HIGH
PERFORMANCE
HEALTH

HiGH PERFORMANCE HEALTH

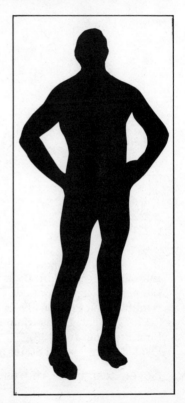

The Revolutionary New Program
For Looking Good, Feeling Good,
And Living A Disease-Free Life

John Yiamouyiannis, Ph.D.

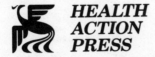

**HEALTH
ACTION
PRESS**

International Standard Book Number: ISBN 0913571-02-4
Library of Congress Catalog Card Number: 87-80031
Health Action Press, 6439 Taggart Road, Delaware, Ohio 43015
©1987 by John Yiamouyiannis. All rights reserved
First Printing: July 1987
Printed in the United States of America

Cover design by Andres A. Caicedo

Contents

Chapter 1

The Promise

Would you like to improve your performance in your business and personal life? Would you like to look younger, feel vibrantly alive, be proud of yourself, your body, and your newfound abilities? Would you like to extend the active and enjoyable period of your life? Would you like to reduce your cancer risk by 90%, develop a strong and healthy heart capable of giving you years of extra service, and avoid other degenerative diseases such as arthritis, gout, osteoporosis, late-onset diabetes, and senility?

If the answer is yes, read on, for what follows opens the doors to the realization of some of your greatest hopes and desires.

When I speak of your health, I am referring to the condition of your body. As the condition of a car, kitchen table, or chair can be good or bad, so can the health of a person be said to be good or bad. The better your health the better you can perform, be active, and do the things which bring happiness. The better your health, the lower the chance you will suffer disease.

You are aware that by taking proper care of your car, you can extend the "life" of your car and also avoid many of the problems that come from neglect. Similarly and more importantly, I am going to show you how to take care of yourself and how, by taking proper care of yourself, you can extend the active and enjoyable period of your life and avoid many of the diseases that come from neglect.

The High Performance Health Program outlined in this book is easy to follow. However, this is not a quick-fix program that you can go on for a few weeks to cure all your ills. (There is virtually nothing that this program can do for you that can't be undone by subsequent abuse.) To be successful, the High Performance Health Program must become a life-style. The guidelines of the program are flexible and encourage variety, making lifetime commitment to the program a pleasure rather than a chore.

The hype and mumbo jumbo of terms such as "scientifically proven", "medically proven", "cure", and "wonder drug" will not be used in the pages of this book. They are either untrue or misleading terms designed to create a medical mystique to justify scandalous profiteering. The only mystique you have to be impressed with is the mystique of your body's abilities to develop, defend, repair, and rejuvenate itself.

Medicine and Science Aren't Mystical

Medicine is nothing more than the art of relieving disease symptoms using methods which bring relatively prompt — yet not necessarily long-lasting — relief, primarily through the use of drugs, appliances, or surgery. While a cure or wonder drug *may* alleviate symptoms or kill germs or cancer cells before it can kill you, sound *lasting* relief will only come when your body kicks in to eliminate the disease. The better your health, the faster this will occur. The better your health, the less chance you will have of getting the disease in the first place.

And there is nothing mystical about science. Science is the observation (by any of the human senses) of physical objects and events and the subsequent classification of these objects and events. Science is important because it brings us the observations and categorizations of events made by many other people and allows us to make conclusions based on their experiences as well as our own.

A Total Program

This book presents a total program that has stood up to observations being made on the frontiers of science. Up to now, health programs have dealt with nutrition *or* exercise *or* environment *or* sleep *or* mental attitude. The few that have dealt with more than one of these factors have dealt with them separately and with little appreciation for their essential interactive effects on health.

For example, a nutritionist might suggest that you increase dietary calcium for stronger bones. However, without anything else being said, this added calcium could settle in your arteries to cause hardening of your arteries, or it could just as well deposit itself in your ligaments, causing arthritis. By means of placing stress on the skeletal system, with progressive weight-lifting work-outs and avoidance of environmental substances, such as fluoride, which stimulate abnormal calcification, this book will explain, among other things, how you can get your body to deposit the calcium you eat into the right places.

Nutritionists tell us "you are what you eat" but many of them are overweight and out of shape. Fitness enthusiasts tell us "No pain, no gain", but they routinely complain about pulled ligaments and tendons, cramps, and more serious irreversible injuries. Environmentalists stress the importance of ridding the environment of substances which are harmful to our health, yet many have little or no knowledge of health. And psychiatrists try to tell us of the importance of proper mental attitude and sleeping habits despite the fact that, as professionals, they have one of the highest suicide rates.

Although each may be aware of a part of the answer, none of them is aware of the total picture. In order for a health program to work, it must deal with all the health factors in an integrated and cohesive manner. The High Performance Health Program does just that.

A Program That Works

The proof is in the pudding. If a program works, it should produce the results that it promises to produce. The High Performance Health Program promises to improve your health, and it does. In addition, it provides the performance tests which directly measure your health and allow you to watch your health improve as you progress through the program. Watching your health improve provides further incentive for you to continue on the program.

To get you to start the program, it might be helpful to relate the experiences of others that have been on the program.

This program was begun over 20 years ago and has been developed and improved during this time. The first person put on the program was my eldest daughter, at birth. In 1984, at the age of 20, she was the first woman in the world, age 21 or under, to cross the finish line in the world-renowned Ironman Triathlon in Hawaii. (This event featured a 2.5-mile swim, 112-mile bike ride, and 26-mile run, nonstop.) Even more astonishing is the fact that she had never in her life run a 26-mile marathon before.

But can this program work in adults? The answer is yes. Any adult who does not have some irreversible disease, such as advanced osteoporosis, that would prevent them from coming on the program, can participate. By conscientiously following the program, people up to the age of 55 or more can reach a performance level higher than an average 20- to 25-year-old. As a participant in this program, at age 44, I can now outperform myself at any other time in my life. For example, at my current weight of 185 pounds, I can now bench press 100 pounds more now than I could at my previous prime as a high school football player when I weighed 216 pounds.

And the program results in dramatically reduced medical costs. Over the course of 20 years, our medical (excluding childbirth) costs have been less than five dollars per person per year, for two adults and six children (aged 13 to 20). Bear in mind that the main thrust of this program is to improve your health, not to teach you how to win in an athletic competition or to save money on medical costs. The program becomes a life-style where winning, looking good, and being disease-free are incidental but welcome symptoms of High Performance Health. The real reward is the feeling of being alive, with blood coursing through your vessels like a raging river rather than sludging around like the contents of some stagnant septic tank. With an improved metabolism and improved oxygen supply to the brain, mental functions become sharper. Your life becomes a life of realization rather than a fantasy of TV soap operas and daydreams.

The Time To Start Is Now

In the spring and early summer of 1985, I took a 5000-mile bicycle trip which brought me to 14 countries in Europe and Africa. One day, as I was cycling through Germany, I ran out of water. I stopped at a home along the way. There was a small outdoor party going on and, as I approached, a man in his late 60s met me. In German, I asked if he could refill my water bottle. The man replied: "It is a great pleasure for me to fill your bottle. I think it's unfortunate that people feel they must wait until some catastrophe occurs before they offer or ask for help."

Probably the number one problem in health care is that people wait for a catastrophe to occur before they start doing something about their health.

On The Program

During this time, you must become selfish. This doesn't mean that you should take the journey by yourself. As a matter of fact, it is advisable to get somebody to get on the program with you. However, whether or not that person drops out, you must be determined to see it through. Sticking with it will pay off not only in an improvement in your health, but a willingness in some of those you love to embark upon the same health improvement program that has led to a more beautiful and vibrant you.

Most important though is that you do this for yourself. And when you have reached the level of high performance health, the journey will not have ended. You will have entered into a new life style of good nutrition, active participation in sports, and a life in an environment more conducive to good health. You will meet others who have taken the same journey and meet new friends. You can take pride in getting others to take the same journey and share with you the new-found joys of your vibrant new life.

Taking Inventory

Get in front of a full length mirror. Take your clothes off. Look at yourself. Are you happy with what you see or glad that you can hide that body underneath clothes? Look yourself over carefully for areas of your body that are excessively fat, underdeveloped. Envision yourself without the excess fat, with muscles (yes, you too, ladies) that are developed. Determine the degree of muscle development you seek.

Make a list of all the diseases you have had. Wouldn't it be nice if you hadn't had to suffer through these diseases? Isn't it nice to know that you can eventually put an end to their recurrence and avoid other diseases that you have not yet experienced?

This book provides a program which nurtures the inherent developmental, defense, repair, and rejuvenation capabilities of your body which can make high performance health and disease-free living a reality for you.

Chapter 2

You and Your Surroundings

Physically, what makes you different from everyone else is your genetics. Your genetics was fully developed within a day after hereditary information from a sperm cell of your father penetrated the egg cell which contained the hereditary information of your mother. Within time, the one fertilized egg cell that was you multiplies to become a body of approximately one hundred trillion (100,000,000,000,000) cells of various shapes and sizes. Whatever your genetic strengths and weaknesses, the state of your health now depends upon the interaction of your body with its surroundings. (Since the terms "surroundings" and "environment" mean exactly the same thing, they will be used interchangeably in this book.)

Your surroundings consist of various physical objects, energies, and forces. By using your senses (sight, hearing, feeling, smelling, and taste), and listening to your body (internal stimulations, pains, hungers, thirsts, desires, etc.), you can learn how to grasp, swallow, breath in, or otherwise expose yourself to factors in your surroundings that nourish (i.e. build up and strengthen) you, and avoid those that can weaken, poison, or demolish you.

Natural Factors That Nourish You

Air	Radio Waves	Infrared Light
Sound	Water	Plants
Temperature	Minerals	Animals
Pressure	Ultraviolet Light	Microorganisms
Gravity	Visible Light	Humans

Nourish, as used in this book, shall be defined as "to promote or stimulate the growth or development of: BUILD UP, STRENGTHEN" [from Webster's Third New International Dictionary (unabridged), 1976]. Natural foods, which are derived from plants, animals, microorganisms or their products and minerals, are thus included in the previous table.

These primary defense mechanisms, i.e. your senses and body signals, are backed up by secondary defense mechanisms. Thus, if you should swallow something harmful, your body has the ability to reject it, digest it, or let it pass through as excrement. If a harmful substance is absorbed into your bloodstream, it can be detoxified by biochemical processes in your body, destroyed by your immune system, or excreted in the urine. If an impact results in bone breakage, your body has the ability to repair the break. Even genetic damage to cells resulting from radiation or chemicals can be repaired by a genetic repair mechanism that exists in every cell of your body.

As remarkable as your body is, problems can arise. Prolonged inadequate nourishment can lead to a breakdown in your body's defense mechanisms and thus to a greater susceptibility to disease. Increased exposure to harmful factors for extended periods can also lead to a breakdown in your defense mechanisms and simultaneously overwork them to cause disease. However, in a natural setting, these problems are relatively easy to avoid.

What complicates matters is that industry, in its attempt to make things which are more convenient and long-lasting — and to make them more easily and profitably — has produced new chemicals and developed new processes to manufacture products (and by-products) that deceive and get past your defense mechanisms like a wolf in sheep's clothing. Thus these chemicals and processes have been used to alter, conceal, color, flavor, pump up, squeeze in, perfume, solidify, liquefy, texturize, extract, fractionate, imitate, capsulize, generate, synthesize, and embalm components in your environment.

As a result, your body is exposed to artificial factors that it was never designed to handle (such as overprocessed foods, artificial food additives, injections, pesticides, toxic chemical by-products, radioactive chemicals, alpha, beta and gamma rays, x-rays, microwaves and ultrasound), as well as concentrations of various natural factors higher than your body was ever designed to handle (such as ultraviolet light, visible light, radio waves, temperature, sound, humans, and various chemicals).

Some Artificially Generated Chemicals That Can Harm You

Water Poisons (inorganic)	Air Poisons (inorganic)	Radioactive Chemicals	Pesticides (organic)
arsenic	hydrogen fluoride	plutonium-239	lindane
cadmium	carbon monoxide	radon-222	aldrin
fluoride	ammonia	radium-226	endrin
mercury	sulfur dioxide	uranium-238	malathion
lead	sulfur trioxide	thorium-232	parathion
barium	nitrogen dioxide	lead-210	heptachlor
beryllium	nitric oxide	samarium-151	dioxins
molybdenum	nitrogen pentoxide	cesium-137	methoxychlor
nickel	ozone	iodine-131	fluoroacetate
chlorine	asbestos dust	strontium-90	DDD
aluminum	silica dust	cobalt-60	2,4-D
tellurium	carbon dust	hydrogen-3	2,4,5-T

Other Air and Water Poisons (organic)		Food Additives	Plastic Foods
formaldehyde	phosgene	sodium benzoate	margarine
benz(a)pyrene	chloroform	formaldehyde	shortening
vinyl chloride	benzene	BHA	hydrogenated oils
methyl isocyanate	PCBs	BHT	processed cheese
trichloroethane	PBBs	MSG	saccharin
β-naphthylamine	acrolein	sorbic acid	cyclamate
acrylonitrile	butadiene	nitrites	aspartame
ethylene chloride	EDB	sulfites	coffee whiteners

This is only a small sample of some of the harmful man-made chemicals. These and other substances will be discussed in Chapter 8. The difference between organic and inorganic is discussed in the Appendix.

In addition, man-made drugs and pain killers have been developed that interfere with your body's ability to function properly and with its ability to provide the signals to let you know what it needs.

A Sample of Notorious Drugs Used

---

thalidomide	bendectin	anabolic steroids	DES
Caragil	valium	chloramphenicol	ibuprofen
swine flu vaccine	Opren	Darvon	imipramine
indomethacin	methyldopa	corticosteroids	Tylenol

For a more detailed discussion of the harmful effects of drugs and how they work, see Chapter 8

The High Performance Health Program will teach you how to recognize, evaluate, and avoid artificial factors that present a threat to your health. The program will also teach you how to use your senses, how to listen to your body, how to select and balance those factors which nourish you, and how to avoid those naturally occurring factors which are harmful. The simplest and best policy is to avoid artificial factors, including drugs. Only in serious health- or life-threatening circumstances should any thought be given to exposing yourself to one of these factors. In these circumstances, you should evaluate the risk of exposure against the possible benefit of the exposure. Such exposures should be short term so that your body is not poisoned long enough to cause irreversible damage. In Chapter 8, I have presented information which will help you in the event you should be faced with making such a decision. The chapters immediately following are designed to help you reduce the chances of finding yourself in serious health- or life-threatening circumstances.

Chapter 3

Getting Started

Y ou are going into this program with a body whose abilities are beyond your wildest dreams. The key to unlocking the immense capabilities of your body is your will. In presenting the High Performance Health Program to you, I merely serve as a tour guide to show you how to unlock, utilize, and protect your body's amazing powers. The fantastic results you will experience will be due to the fact that you thought enough of yourself to take the time, energy, and money necessary to begin the program and stick with it. Your body will do the rest.

How much are you worth to yourself? Christians refer to the body as the temple of the Holy Spirit. Yet, looking at them reveals that many have forsaken the temple. And what about you? Are you willing to spend $10,000 to $25,000 or more for a car and additional thousands each year to maintain it and yet begrudge spending a small portion of your time and money to get your body in good shape and keep it there?

The average person 18 years or over spends 32 hours a week watching television. Don't tell me that they can't find 3-4 hours a week to do the core activities of the High Performance Health Program. And don't tell me that they can't spend some of the remaining 27-28 hours of this time with more worthwhile recreational activities such as bicycling, dancing, sailing, skiing, swimming, and tennis. They can find the time and so can you.

The Program

Whether you are athletic or out of shape, this program is designed to improve your performance and bring your health to a high performance health level. If you are out of shape, the program will put you "in shape".

Notice that I emphasize body shape and do not refer to body weight. Body weight is composed of two major divisions, body fat and lean body mass. Among other things, this program is designed to decrease body fat levels and increase lean body mass by increasing muscle mass and to a lesser extent, bone mass.

To start the program, get in front of a mirror with your clothes off and take a look at yourself. Regardless of what your total weight is, if your body fat percentage is high, you will not be pleased with what you see. Taking a picture of yourself in a revealing bathing suit, both head-on and side-view now and at monthly intervals, will be helpful in tracking your progress as you go through the program. However, make sure that you take and record measurements of yourself in the following areas right now, and each month hereafter.

	now	1	2	3	4	5	6
Chest (relaxed)							
Chest (expanded)							
Waist (relaxed)							
Waist (pulled in)							
Hips							
Thigh							
Calf							
Biceps (relaxed)							
Biceps (flexed)							
Forearm (relaxed)							
Forearm (flexed)							

Measurements can be made most easily with a cloth tape measure. You will also find that it is easier (and possibly more fun) if you have someone else take your measurements. If you are out of shape, when you start the program, the results as you continue on the program will be dramatic. Comparing these measurements with your monthly pictures will give you objective evidence to show you that what you are seeing is really happening.

By itself, weight is not a good way to track your progress as you go through the program. In combination with the above measurements however, it can give you a preliminary idea of how you are doing. That is, if you are putting inches on or taking them off in the right places, weight changes will tip you off before you can see noticeable changes in your body measurements.

You can get a better indication of how you are progressing by watching changes in your body fat. Ideally, these measurements should be made the first, third, and sixth months into the program. Many spas can provide you with an approximate estimate of your body fat using the caliper method or the conductivity method. However, if you are serious about getting an accurate measurement of your body fat, contact the exercise physiology department or the athletic department at your local state university and ask them where you can get your body fat determined by the immersion method. **Under no circumstances should you delay going on or continuing with the program because you haven't had your body fat measured.**

	NOW	1	2	3	4	5	6
Weight	___	___	___	___	___	___	___
% Body Fat	___			___			___
Weight of Body Fat	___			___			___
Lean Body Weight	___			___			___

Once you have your weight and your % body fat measurement you can calculate the weight of your body fat and your lean body weight. For example, if you weigh 150 pounds and your body fat is 35%, you multiply 150 X 35/100 which equals 52.5 pounds. You then subtract the 52.5 pounds from the 150 pounds and find that you have a lean body weight of 97.5 pounds. These calculations can easily be done for you by the person taking your body fat measurements.

The goal for men should be to get their body fat below 15%, but no lower than 4-6%. Women should try to get their body fat below 18%, but no lower than 6-8%.

In the above example, if the person is a female, 5 feet 5 inches tall, she might reasonably expect to reach a high performance health level at a weight of 130 pounds and a body fat percentage of 15%. That means that her target body fat weight would be 19.5 pounds (i.e. 135 X 15/100) and her target lean body weight would be 110.5 pounds. This means she must lose 33 pounds of fat and put on 13 pounds of lean body weight, mostly in the form of muscle.

In the above example, if the person is a male, 5 feet 8 inches tall, he might reasonably expect to reach a high performance health level at a weight of 170 pounds and a body fat percentage of 10%. That means that his target body fat weight would be 17 pounds (i.e. 170 X 10/100) and his target lean body weight would be 153 pounds. This means he must lose 25.5 pounds of fat and put on 55.5 pounds of lean body weight, mostly in the form of muscle.

In order to bring about these changes, a carefully designed exercise program integrated with a sophisticated diet, proper rest periods for recovery, an awareness of factors to stay away from, and most importantly a positive mental attitude is required.

Chapter 4

An Integrated Approach
Doing What Your Physician Can't

Humpty Dumpty sat on the wall
Humpty Dumpty had a great fall
All the King's horses and all the King's men
Couldn't put Humpty together again

The key to the High Performance Health Program is that it is an integrated approach. No matter how good your current eating habits are, if you do not engage in an adequate amount of activity, it will be virtually impossible for you to get the proper amount of each of the food components you need to keep your body functioning properly. This is in part due to the fact that it is difficult to get the substances necessary for the proper functioning of your body in your caloric budget without an adequate amount of activity. Your caloric budget is determined by the amount of energy you expend. If you take in more energy than you put out, you alter your body shape and composition so that you cannot perform properly. If you cut down on the amount of energy you take in, you may keep your weight steady, but you will not get enough of the food components necessary for your body to function as it should.

Furthermore, physical activity itself serves to create the demand needed to tell your body where to deposit food components and what to do with them. It provides a stimulus for using the food components you take in to form strong bones, ligaments, tendons, and cartilage. It stimulates the formation of muscles capable of providing greater energy output. It keeps the metabolic processes of your body going allowing your body to produce hormones, and allowing your body's developmental, defense, repair, and rejuvenation capabilities to do their job.

On the other hand, it is obvious that no matter how good your fitness program is, you will not perform well unless your eating habits are good. The foods you eat provide the raw materials to supply you with energy and make the products necessary to keep your body functioning properly. So, no matter how good your physical activity program is, if you do not have a good nutritional program, you will not have the proper raw materials or energy-producing ingredients to keep your body performing properly.

In short, food supplies energy and raw materials to your body. Physical activity uses energy to perform tasks and stimulate the proper utilization of raw materials in your body. As activity levels change, so do your body's food requirements. Without knowing what your activity levels are, it is senseless for anyone to suggest to you how much of each food to eat. Similarly, without supplying you with the proper nutrition, it is difficult for someone to get you to perform well physically.

Thus, you may have been very conscientious in following a good diet *or* fitness program and still not be experiencing good health because you have been neglecting the other. One other warning I should offer at this point is that **no matter how conscientious you have been with your diet or fitness programs, do not skip these sections of the book.** I assure you that, while they may start off in an elementary fashion for clarity, the most advanced student of diet or fitness will pick up vital information in these sections. Furthermore, the incorporation of both these disciplines into an integrated approach will require that you have followed them in the course of this book.

Good health can escape even those who follow the nutritional and fitness guidelines outlined in this book. Other environmental factors which are harmful and do not nurture the body can undo the constructive changes brought about by a good dietary and fitness program. Thus, this book incorporates into the program the means by which you can recognize and avoid those substances in your environment which are harmful to your health.

Sleep is also an important part of the High Performance Health Program. After having balanced all the other health factors, sound sleep should come as a natural result. While you can mentally interfere with your body's ability to sleep, I advise you not to. Sound sleep allows your body to spend most of its attention in repairing, recuperating, rejuvenating, and developing itself. In general, you should allow yourself 7-9 hours of sleep each night (even more is necessary for young children). Inadequate sleep will show up in your inability to perform well on the performance tests outlined in this book.

Bodies which are in good health thrive on extremes. If you engage in vigorous activities regularly, you will tend to feel more wide awake and alert during your active hours and you will tend to be a sound sleeper and more rested after your resting hours. In contrast, if you work at a desk job and your after-work activities include nothing more exerting than lying down in front of the TV set, you will tend to be a lighter sleeper. In this case, the difference between sleep and wakefulness become a monotonous blur from which there appears to be no escape.

This can also be seen by looking at heart rate. If you are active and on a good diet, you will be more able to increase your heart beat (through activity) for a sustained period of time and yet, while you are at rest, you will have a resting heart rate below that of an inactive person. If you are inactive you will never have the performance capabilities of an active person since, among other reasons, you can't sustain an increased heart rate. In addition, your resting heart rate will be higher. Again, the difference between maximum and minimum heart rate is much greater for people in a high performance health condition than for people who lead a sedentary life.

The lust of life for extremes (intense activity and intense rest) also affects other vital health attributes such as the strength, vitality, and youthfulness of bones, joints, ligaments, tendons, muscles, blood, and virtually every system in the body. In a natural setting, this lust is supported by the need to survive. In a "civilized" setting, a strong mental attitude is necessary to push you to do the things necessary to keep yourself in high performance health condition. The alternative to pushing yourself physically in the civilized setting, while not as clear as in the natural setting, can nevertheless be seen in the slow degeneration of the bodies of those who choose not to. Go to an old age home. Watch an Alzheimers patient. See someone with osteoporosis in the prime of their life. Commiserate with those who are cut down or incapacitated with a whole life ahead of them. Youth often gives the false assurance that you can coast through life without ill-health knocking at your door. Don't wait.

Performance testing gives you the early warning system to let you know that your health is beginning to deteriorate before disease hits you over the head (sometimes with a fatal blow) to assure you that something is wrong. The High Performance Health Program gives you the means for stopping these diseases before they start.

How many people have gone to their physician and passed their physicals with flying colors only to find out at their next physical six months later that they have cancer. "But doctor, six months ago, you said I was in excellent health. Now you say I have cancer." It is tragic but true that physicians, while experts with disease, are generally so out-of-touch with health that they cannot predict a disease before it has afflicted their patients. Even more shocking and revealing is the fact that even if your physician were able to tell you that you were going to get cancer over the next six months, he/she wouldn't be able to tell you how to avoid it.

Chapter 5

Getting The Things You Need

In nature, air, water, minerals, plants, and animals provide you with all the nutrients you need to develop, build up and strengthen your body.

Of these, oxygen is the most important, though most overlooked nutrient. Depending on how active you are, you will use between 1 and 4 pounds of it each day. If deprived of oxygen for from 2 to 30 minutes, you will die.

Water is the next most important nutrient. Depending on how active you are, you will use 3 to 8 pounds of it each day. If deprived of water for from 4 to 15 days, you will die.

Together with air and water, minerals and light provide the only nutrients necessary to make most plants grow. Plants use minerals, water and carbon dioxide from the air, and sunlight to form hundreds of thousands of chemicals which we commonly refer to as food. Animals as well as other plants (e.g. mushrooms) use this food for nourishment. Humans use foods derived from plants as well as animals (e.g. human mother's milk) for nourishment. Exposure to any other chemicals for nourishment is an invitation to health problems.

How to get good oxygen

Oxygen is the hardest nutrient to obtain in a noncontaminated form. The best measure you can take to improve the quality of the air you breathe is to live in a rural area. By doing this, you can get away from the carbon monoxide, sulfur dioxide, nitrogen oxides, incompletely combusted petroleum products, lead, and other health-threatening substances that exist in the air of various urban areas as a result of specific industries. Even those of you who live in the country can be subjected to the poisoning of your air by heavy industries located nearby (such as phosphate fertilizer plants, metal foundries, power-generating facilities, and certain petrochemical plants) as well as by the intensive spraying of agricultural areas. However, by living in rural areas selected with an eye out for surrounding industries and the pesticide-spraying practices of the area, you can find relatively clean sources of oxygen.

> *Of the 100 U.S. counties having the highest lung cancer rates between 1950 and 1970, 50 were in the states of Texas, Louisiana, Mississippi, Alabama, and Tennessee, most of which form a continuous band from Houston to Mobile, and up the Mississippi River to Memphis. Of the remaining high lung-cancer counties, 25 are in Florida, Georgia, and South Carolina, 13 are in Maryland, Virginia, and North Carolina, and 5 are in New Jersey and adjacent areas (Philadelphia and Western Long Island). Many of these areas are known for their petrochemical and phosphate fertilizer industries; some of these counties are also in metal foundry areas. Two contiguous counties in Montana (Deer Lodge and Silver Bow), which are also among these high lung cancer counties, are in the midst of the large Anaconda metal foundry area. Only 5 of the 100 highest lung cancer counties lie outside the areas listed above.*

If the term "poisoning of your air" seems too harsh a term to use and you feel that pollution would be a more suitable word, I suggest you consider the following definitions obtained from Webster's Dictionary. The term environmental pollution is not only inappropriate but it also covers up the seriousness of the problem we are dealing with. It has been used to describe what is, in fact, the poisoning of our surroundings. A true understanding of – and an incentive to do something about – this very serious situation cannot come about until we recognize that we are being poisoned by ourselves and the industries that are dumping harmful chemicals into our surroundings, including the air we breathe, the water we drink, and the food we eat.

Poison — a substance that in suitable quantity has properties harmful or fatal to an organism . . .

Poison — to give poison to: to kill or injure by means of a poison, to put poison on or into, to taint, impregnate or infect with poison

Poisoning — the abnormal condition produced by a poisonous or toxic substance

Pollution — emission of semen (sperm) at other times than in coition (sexual intercourse)

From Webster's Third New International Dictionary (unabridged), 1976

If you live in an urban area, the best bet is to live where there is little or no heavy industry. If there is heavy industry, the only alternative you have is to get politically active to make sure that these industries (such as the aluminum, phosphate, power-generating, steel, and petrochemical industries) have devices that will remove as much of the poisons that they are throwing into the air (such as fluorides, sulfur dioxide, and benz(a)pyrene) as current technology allows and, if current technology cannot cope with the problem, to shut down the industry (this has the surprising effect of inducing the rapid "advancement of current technology" in these areas).

If the power-generating plant near you is a nuclear facility, there is little current technology can do to stop the day-to-day poisoning of the air by radioisotopes, such as tritium (hydrogen-3), which can cause cancer and birth defects. This is one of the reasons that a number of politically active groups are campaigning against nuclear power plants, which put out toxic products in a form which is not offensive to the eye or the nose but which poison us nonetheless (see Chapter 8).

The problems of automobile exhausts and other persistent poisonous chemicals that cannot be properly controlled make urban living a second class choice at best if your health is a priority issue with you. For example, in an urban setting, your chances of dying of lung cancer are about twice as great than if you live in a rural setting.

Area	Years	Lung Cancer Death Rate[1] (for white males)
Rural areas of rural states[2]	1950-1970	22
25 largest cities[3]	1950-1970	47

[1]the number of white males dying each year of lung cancer per 100,000 white males in the population
[2]North Dakota, South Dakota, Idaho, Montana, New Mexico, Wyoming
[3]New York City, Chicago, Los Angeles, Philadelphia, Detroit, Baltimore, Houston, Cleveland, Washington DC, Boston, Milwaukee, St. Louis, San Francisco, Dallas, Pittsburgh, Buffalo, New Orleans, San Antonio, San Diego, Seattle Cincinnati, Atlanta, Kansas City, Newark

Deaths from other causes are also considerably greater in urban areas. This is due not only to air quality but also to items like increased stress from the fast pace, increased noise levels, traffic, and sedentary life-style, that are associated with urban living.

Chemicals in the air at your work place and in your home can present a hazard in addition to the poisoning of the outside air. Use your nose. If you smell something, find out where it is coming from. If you find that it is some harmful substance, such as a solvent, cigaret smoke, a cleaning agent, a petroleum product, a pesticide, etc., see what you can do to keep it out of the air you breathe. If you must use poisonous chemicals such as ammonia and chlorine bleach in your home, make sure you have adequate ventilation. Open up your windows. Similarly, if you are using paint removers or other solvents, make sure the area is well ventilated and get the job done as

quickly as possible. Try to eliminate or keep the use of poisonous chemicals to a minimum. If you smell gas fumes in your
house or smell fuel oil, get the problem solved as soon as possible. Certainly, don't let anyone, including yourself, smoke in
your home.

How to get good water

> *"In a world context the most effective general health
> measure would be the provision of adequate clean
> water."*
>
> from *Cured to Death* by
> Arabella Melville and Colin Johnson

In contrast to air, water is fairly easy to get in a non-contami-
nated form. With few exceptions, a home water distiller with
a solid-block charcoal prefilter will remove contaminants from
your drinking water. [see Appendix] You can also purchase
distilled water from the grocery store or have it delivered to
your home by a bottled water company. If you should prefer to
buy or use spring water or well water instead, consider that
some waters that are sold have been shown to have very high
levels of poisonous chemicals in them. This is not to say that
there are not some good spring waters and well waters available, but if you use these waters, you should get a complete
analysis of the water and then have the analysis evaluated.
[see Appendix]

If you are concerned about the fact that distilled water lacks
minerals and that use of it may deplete the body of minerals,
I should stress that water is not a reliable source for minerals.
In some cases, water may contain high magnesium/low calcium; in other areas it may contain low magnesium/high calcium or low magnesium/low calcium/high sodium or high arse-
nic/high fluoride/high sodium. In order to receive a proper
amount and balance of minerals, one must rely on a diet
composed of fresh fruits and vegetables (which themselves
supply you with a significant amount of water) as well as nuts,
seeds, and other natural products, which have preselected

those minerals in proportions necessary for the proper maintenance of life.

Once you have started using distilled water or a reliable spring water or well water, you should use it not only for drinking, but also for the dilution of concentrated fruit juices and any other liquid which you or anyone in your family might consume that requires the addition of water. It also should be used in the preparation of foods such as rice, spaghetti, cooked cereals, beans, soups, bread, and sprouts, which take up substantial amounts of water when prepared.

How to get good food

While modern supermarkets are loaded with junk foods, they still carry a large number of very good foods. Most of the good foods are located around the perimeter of the store with a few located in the aisles.

Walking through a supermarket in a small midwestern town in early March, I was able to find the following first class foods:

Fresh Raw Vegetables

mung bean sprouts	sweet potatoes	leaf lettuce	eggplant
spaghetti squash	sweet peppers	red lettuce	potatoes
Brussels sprouts	yellow squash	asparagus	zucchini
Chinese cabbage	acorn squash	rutabaga	radishes
romaine lettuce	hot peppers	parsnips	carrots
alfalfa sprouts	red cabbage	broccoli	parsley
iceberg lettuce	cauliflower	escarole	cabbage
Boston lettuce	green beans	bok choy	turnips
spinach	tomato	endive	chives
onions	garlic	celery	

Selection will vary with the time of the year and region of the country.

Fresh Raw Fruits

honeydew melon	tangerines	nectarines	apple
bananas	watermelon	oranges	peaches
pears	grapes	cantaloupe	lemon
plums	pineapple	avocados	grapefruit
lime			

Selection will vary with the time of the year and region of the country.

Raw Nuts

walnuts	brazil nuts	hazelnuts	almonds
peanuts	black walnuts	pecans	pine nuts
coconuts			

Food "co-ops" and health food stores often have a wider selection of raw nuts. In this town, I found that the local co-op carried all of the above raw nuts plus raw cashews.

Fresh Raw Meats

beef	pork	lamb	ocean perch
salmon	swordfish	monkfish	catfish
turkey	chicken	scallops	oysters
whitefish	flounder	shrimp	clams
mahi mahi	amberjack	haddock	scrod
Boston blue	whitefish	shark	cod
sole			

Avoid cured hams, bacons, cold cuts, hotdogs, or other processed meats. If you insist on eating them, at least be sure that they are labeled so that you can be sure that you want to eat everything they contain. Do not eat them if they contain artificial additives such as sodium nitrite. When buying fresh meat, it is preferable, to buy whole pieces. For example, when buying a chicken, buy a whole chicken rather than chicken parts. That way you know what the whole animal looked like and can be sure the best parts of two or three rotting chickens weren't thrown together to make up a "chicken". Similarly, it is best to buy beef in solid pieces rather than ground. Grinding beef ahead of time increases the spoilage rate of meat. Most good supermarkets will have a butcher who will cut up your chicken or grind your beef for you.

Fresh Organs

chicken liver   lamb liver   chicken   gizzard

Fresh Eggs

chicken eggs

Dried Beans

limas   pintos   kidney   pea
Great Northern   black-eyes   lentils

Food "co-ops" and health food stores often have a wider selection of beans. In this town, I found that the local co-op carried all of the above beans plus the following: adzuki, black, garbanzos, red lentils, mung, navy, and yellow pea.

Dry Cereals and Seeds

oatmeal (old fashioned)   brown rice
cracked wheat   whole rye flour
whole cornmeal (undegerminated)   pearl barley
popcorn   sunflower seeds
wheat flour

Food "co-ops" and health food stores often have a wider selection of cereals and seeds. In this town, I found that the local co-op carried all of the above cereals and seeds plus the following: buckwheat, millet, alfalfa, pumpkin seeds, and sesame seeds.

Spice Seeds

black pepper   white pepper   mustard seed   dill seed
nutmeg   allspice   cardammon   anise
carraway seed   sesame seed   poppy seed   cumin
celery seed   fennel seed

The above spice seeds can be purchased whole or ground. Freshly grinding the seeds immediately before use is recommended. While these spices do not comprise a large part of your diet, what little nutrition they do provide is good; they also provide a natural source for food flavoring.

In this supermarket, I was also able to find the following second class foods. While not as good as the above foods, they may still find an occasional purpose for being in your diet.

Frozen Vegetables

green beans	corn	lima beans	asparagus
peas	Brussels sprouts	broccoli	cauliflower
carrots			

If fresh vegetables do not provide enough variety for you, go with frozen rather than canned vegetables.

Frozen Fruits

strawberries	blueberries	raspberries	cherries
blackberries			

Fresh fruits are preferable however since berries have such a short season, it is often nice to use frozen berries to add variety to your fruit selection.

Juices

orange juice　apple juice　grapefruit juice　　pineapple juice

Juices made from fresh raw fruits and vegetables just before serving are the best and the variety is broad.

When buying bottled juices, make sure that the juice is in a glass bottle or a cardboard carton. Lead contamination from fruit juices from the solder of cans has been a problem leading to arthritis, among other problems. Also make sure that the juice is not from concentrate for two reasons: (1) concentration and redilution are two more processing steps which reduce the nutritional value of the product and (2) you do not know what kind of water was used to redilute the concentrate. You are better off buying frozen concentrated juice (orange, apple, grapefruit, or pineapple and diluting it with distilled water). Virtually all frozen concentrated grape juices contain added sugar and should be avoided.

At this supermarket, the only suitable bottled orange juice I could find was Tropicana orange juice, pure premium (white carton). This juice is not from concentrate and is the best prepackaged orange juice that I am aware of. (In some other supermarkets, I have seen freshly squeezed orange juice in the produce sections.) For apple juice, insist upon unsweetened (preferably unfiltered) apple juice in jars, not from concentrate. At this supermarket I found two brands, Mott's and Speas, that were satisfactory.

You may increase your variety by putting a handful of frozen unsweetened berries such as strawberries, blueberries, raspberries, blackberries, or cherries into a blender half-filled with apple juice and blending them for about 5-10 seconds. This will add another 5 or so flavors to your juice list. By itself, or with the addition of ice or distilled water to this recipe, you have a drink in addition to the other juices with which to wean yourself and your children away from soft drinks.

In addition to the juices listed above, food "co-ops" and health food stores often have pineapple juice, grape juice, tomato juice, and carrot juice which are not made from concentrate and which are packaged in glass bottles.

By all means stay away from juices that contain additives such as potassium sorbate, sulfur dioxide, sulfites, and benzoates. Also be sure to stay away from fruit drinks, such as Hawaiian Punch, Hi-C, Gator Aid, Kool Aids, etc. that may have a fruit-like flavor but are loaded with added white sugar.

Salted and/or Roasted Nuts and Seeds

peanuts   cashews   macadamia nuts
pistacho nuts   sunflower seeds

Stay away from "honey" roasted nuts. The primary sweetener in these nuts is sugar or some cheap corn sweetener.

Nut Butters

peanut butter

When buying peanut butter in the supermarket, buy the natural, salted or unsalted. Food "co-ops" and health food stores often have a wider selection of nut butters. In this town, I found that the local co-op carried all of the above nut butters plus cashew butter, sesame butter (tahini), and almond butter.

Fats

unsalted sweetcream butter   virgin (cold pressed) olive oil
salted sweetcream butter   lard (without additives)

Food "co-ops" and health food stores often have a wider selection of suitable fats. In this town, I found that the local co-op carried all of the above fats (excluding lard) plus the following: cold-pressed peanut oil, cold-pressed corn oil, cold-pressed almond oil, cold-pressed coconut oil, and cold-pressed palm kernel oil. Other oils available in the supermarket are not cold-pressed and as result, during the harsher extraction process, many of the nutritionally important components are lost.

Be sure that whenever you buy a fat to stay away from margarine, vegetable shortening, or partially hydrogenated oil, as well as any oil or fat containing preservatives such as BHA and BHT.

Frozen Meats

cornish hen	perch	tuna	turkey
crabmeat	lobster tail	duck	lox
orange roughy	catfish	frog legs	cod
sole	snapper	shrimp	

While not as good as fresh meats, frozen meats add more variety to your diet.

Spice Vegetables (Dried)

sweet basil	oregano	tarragon	chervil
sage	marjoram	savory	thyme
saffron	garlic	bay leaves	rosemary
dill weed	cinnamon	cloves	orange peel
lemon rind	hot pepper	chives	ginger
horseradish	paprika	green onions	onion
parsley			

The spice vegetables that are available fresh, such as green onions, onions, parsley, and garlic, should be purchased fresh. Since the others are eaten in such small quantities, using them in the dehydrated state will not seriously affect your diet.

Dry Fruit

prunes	raisins	coconut	dates

While dried apricots, pineapple, peaches, and mixed fruit were also available, they each had added sulfites and/or sugar added and thus should be avoided. It must be remembered that dry fruits are, at best, a poor substitute for fresh fruits. As an alternative to candies and sweets, however, they are the better choice.

Sweeteners

frozen concentrated juices   honey
molasses   maple syrup

The characteristic flavor of each of these sweeteners makes their use self-limiting. While you can add tremendous amounts of sugar to something without altering the taste very much, if you add very much of any of the above sweeteners, you will destroy the taste of the food you were trying to sweeten by overpowering it with the taste of the sweetener.

Unlike sugar, these sweeteners have nutritional value beyond the nutritional value of the sugar which makes up their bulk. In addition, rather than containing one sugar, they contain a number of different sugars. For example, in addition to the fructose, glucose, and sucrose found in other refined sugar sweeteners, honey contains the following natural sugars: glucose 6-phosphate, maltose, isomaltose, nigerose, turanose, maltulose, kojibiose, neotrehalose, gentiobiose, laminaribiose, t-kestose, melezitose, 6^G-α-glucosylsucrose, panose, isomaltotriose, erlose, 3-α-isomaltosylglucose, isopanose, isomaltotetraose, isomaltopentaose, and centose, as well as other natural substances such as α- or β-glycerophosphate, 2- or 3-phosphoglyceric acid, lactic acid, pyruvic acid, α-ketoglutaric acid, citric acid, acetic acid, butyric acid, formic acid, gluconic acid, malic acid, maleic acid, oxalic acid, pyroglutamic acid, succinic acid, glycollic acid, tartaric acid, arabogalactomannan, proteins, nucleoproteins, enzymes, and trace amounts of vitamins, as well as the following minerals: potassium, sodium, calcium, magnesium, iron, copper, manganese, chloride, phosphorus, sulfur, silica, chromium, and others.

By all means stay away from artificial sweeteners such as aspartame, (alias Nutrisweet), sacccharin, and cyclamate.

Sodium Salts

table salt (sodium chloride)
baking soda (sodium bicarbonate)
baking powder   (sodium bicarbonate, calcium acid phosphate, cornstarch)

When choosing table salt or baking powder, avoid additives such as sodium silicoaluminate (sodium aluminum silicate), potassium iodide ("iodine"), dextrose (sugar), or any other additive. Table salt or baking powder without these additives can usually be purchased at a health food store or a food co-op. Sometimes cream of tartar (tartaric acid) is used in place of calcium acid phosphate. The use of all these salts should be limited because they are extremely high in sodium. However, since the High Performance Health Program requires a higher level of activity, moderate use of these salts should not present a problem after being on the program for a month. Unnecessary use of baking soda, such as its use in keeping vegetables looking green should be discouraged since it will tend to destroy the vitamin value of vegetables.

Miscellaneous Foods

vinegar   prepared mustard   tamari   baker's yeast

Experiment by substituting freshly squeezed lemon juice for vinegar in some of your recipes. When buying vinegar, stay away from distilled vinegar. The prepared mustard you buy should contain vinegar, mustard, and salt. If it contains other ingredients, make sure that there is no sugar or artificial additive added. Tamari is a suitable alternative to soy sauce, which almost always contains sodium benzoate. Usually not available at supermarkets, tamari can be purchased at health food stores and food co-ops.

Milks and Creams

sour cream	milk	buttermilk
yoghurt	cream	

Ideally, these products should not be in your diet. While they do provide useful nutrients to the body, they have an adverse effect on performance and tend to sludge the body down. Some people can't handle milk sugar (lactose) properly while others have a problem with milk protein (which often is a problem with cheeses). Consumption of these products leads to increased mucus production and allergies in a surprising number of people.

If you do decide to drink milk, sip it, don't gulp it. If you sip it, milk will curdle in the form of fine strands when it hits the acid in the stomach and these fine strands can be digested easily. If you gulp it, milk will curdle in the form of golf-balls, some of which will pass through the stomach and a portion of the intestines, sludging up the intestines along the way.

Milk processors have added other reasons why milk should not be consumed: (1) they have pasteurized it and – as a result – have denatured milk proteins, giving rise to proteins which may be less digestible or more likely to produce allergies; (2) they have homogenized it to produce a suspension of fine fat droplets in milk and researchers are now reporting that as a result, these minute fat droplets encapsulate an enzyme (xanthine oxidase) and carry that enzyme through the intestinal wall into the bloodstream where it can cause damage; (3) they have ultrapasteurized cream in an attempt to give it a longer shelf life, producing enough damage to the product to give it a slightly scalded taste (ultrapasteurization is a process which heats products to an extremely high temperature for short periods of time); (4) they have literally "skimmed the cream" off your milk telling you how much better off you are with low fat milk, then taking the cream and selling this same fat to you directly at a higher price or churning the fat out of the cream into butter (which is 89% milk fat) and again selling it to you at a higher price (Ironically, milk fat does not have any of the adverse effects that milk sugar or milk protein have.); (5) they have added synthetic vitamin D (irradiated ergosterol), which may have harmful side-effects, to milk.

Even certified raw milk, which is not generally available, produces some of the intolerances discussed above. Raw goat's milk, which is not readily available, is less allergenic and is often given to infants who cannot handle cow's milk. Human mother's milk is obviously the milk of choice for humans.

Natural Cheeses

Monterey Jack	Cheddar	brick	Colby
farmers	Romano	parmesan	feta
Edam	blue	Mozzarella	havarti
pepper	gouda	Muenster	butter cheese
provolone	cream		

Stay away from any cheese that has an orange tint or color and stay away from all "processed" cheeses, such as Velveeta and American. Also, see the warning under "milks and creams". Remember, the milk protein in cheese has already been curdled during the cheese-making process so the curdling problems that exist with milk do not exist with cheese.

If the above categories of foods do not seem to be enough variety for you, let's take a look at what's available on the shelves in the aisles of the supermarket. About 17% of the shelf space is taken up by nonedible items such as soaps, detergents, cleaning aids, paper goods, bags, tobacco products, etc. Pet foods take up about 4%. Of the remaining space, about 54% is taken up by foods loaded with sugar and white flour with artificial color and flavoring added to fool you into thinking that you are getting variety in your diet when in fact all you are getting are calories devoid or nearly devoid of the vitamins, minerals, and other growth factors necessary for good health. Such "foods" include candies, cookies, cake, cookie, and frosting mixes, juice drinks, Kool Aid-type drinks and gelatin desserts, sugar-laden "ready-to-eat" cereals, soda pop, jams and jellies, puddings and pie fillings, sugars and corn syrups, ice creams and sherbets, etc. In short, over 50% of the food shelf space is taken up by foods whose primary ingredients are sugar and/or white flour. Not very much variety. About 38% of the food shelf space is taken up by items such as potato chips, frozen prepared meals and TV-type dinners, canned goods, and other seminutritious items such as catsup, which contains about 30-40% added sugar. Only about 8% of the food shelf space is taken up by the foods on the recommended list.

Most of these foods are found along the perimeter of the store in the produce and meat sections.

Foods to Stay Away From

	Reason				
Food	Contains Too much Refined Sugar[1]	Contains Too much Refined Flour[2]	Contains Trash Fats	Contains Artificial Colors & Flavors	Contains Other Harmful Additives
cold cereals	yes	yes	no	maybe	maybe
cookies	yes	yes	yes	maybe	maybe
breads and rolls	some	yes	yes	maybe	maybe
frozen cakes	yes	yes	yes	maybe	maybe
breakfast bars	yes	yes	yes	yes	maybe
jellos	yes	no	no	yes	maybe
puddings	yes	no[3]	no	yes	maybe
pie fillings	yes	no[3]	no	maybe	maybe
frostings	yes	yes	yes	yes	maybe
sugar	yes	no	no	no	no
corn syrups	yes	no	no	no	no

Foods to Stay Away From (Continued)

Food	Contains Too much Refined Sugar[1]	Contains Too much Refined Flour[2]	Contains Trash Fats	Contains Artificial Colors & Flavors	Contains Other Harmful Additives
			Reason		
imitation maple syrup	yes	no	no	yes	maybe
marshmallows	yes	no[3]	no	yes	maybe
soda pop	yes	no	no	yes	maybe
juice drinks	yes	no	no	yes	maybe
juice flavored drinks	yes	no	no	yes	maybe
sherbets	yes	no	no	yes	maybe
ice cream	yes	no	maybe	yes	maybe
candy	yes	no	maybe	yes	maybe
jams	yes	no	no	maybe	maybe
jellies	yes	no	no	maybe	maybe
cocoa mixes	yes	no	maybe	yes	maybe
chip dips	maybe	no[3]	yes	yes	maybe
pickles	maybe	no	yes	yes	maybe
catsup	yes	no	no	no	no
soy sauces	some	yes	no	maybe	maybe
potato chips	no	no	yes	no	maybe
corn chips	no	no	yes	no	maybe
pretzels	maybe	yes	yes	no	maybe
toritos	no	no	yes	no	maybe
premade popcorn	no	no	yes	no	maybe
cheese curls[4]	no	no	yes	no	maybe
salad dressings	some	no	yes	maybe[5]	maybe
mayonnaises	some	no	yes	maybe	maybe
popping oils	no	no	yes	yes	maybe
margarine	no	no	yes	yes	maybe
shortening	no	no	yes	yes	maybe
hydrogenated oil	no	no	yes	yes	maybe
imitation creams	yes	no	yes	yes	maybe

Foods to Stay Away From (Continued)

Food	Contains Too much Refined Sugar[1]	Contains Too much Refined Flour[2]	Contains Trash Fats	Contains Artificial Colors & Flavors	Contains Other Harmful Additives
			Reason		
artificial whipped creams	yes	no	yes	yes	maybe
crackers	no	yes	yes	maybe	maybe
muffin, cookie and cake mixes	yes	yes	yes	maybe	maybe

[1]refined sugar refers to white sugar, corn syrup, dextrose, glucose, fructose, corn sweeteners, and other highly refined sugars that do not provide any other nutritional value.
[2]refined flour refers to refined flours derived from wheat (except in the case of cold cereals and breakfast bars which may contain the refined products of other grains)
[3]while these products do not contain white flour, they sometimes contain cornstarch which, like white flour, provides virtually no nutritional value other than calories.
[4]also includes products such as bugles and pringles.
[5]rarely, mainly in Weightwatchers products.

Foods That Contain Too Much Refined Sugar

Your ancestors in the caveman days could burn up to 7000-8000 calories each day. The very sedentary lifestyles of modern man have reduced the number of calories of food that can be consumed without becoming fat to as low as 2000 or less. Working with a caloric budget of only 25% of our ancestors' budget, it is almost impossible to get enough of the nutrients necessary to develop, strengthen, and build up your body on the average American diet. While the High Performance Health Program will increase your total caloric budget by increasing your level of activity, you must make your calories count. You cannot afford to spend calories from this limited caloric budget on foods such as refined sugars (sucrose, glucose or dextrose, or fructose), which are high in calories and contain *none* of the vitamins, minerals, and other essential factors necessary for good health. This means that you must avoid foods which are made with refined sugars.

If you are like the average American, you consume about one teaspoon of sugar every half hour, 24 hours a day! That translates into 48 teaspoons of sugar per day. While this may seem like an impossible amount, when you consider that a can of cola contains about 10 teaspoons of added white sugar — or when you consider that every heaping teaspoon of ice cream contains a level teaspoon of added white sugar — or when you consider that many of the above "foods", such as candies, cookies, cakes, gelatin desserts, sugar-laden "ready-to-eat" cereals, jams, jellies, and puddings contain more than 50% added white sugar — and when you consider that even foods you would never expect to find sugar in, such as catsup, salad dressings, mayonnaises, bread, pickles, soy sauce, pretzels, and even salt, contain added white sugar, you can see that it is not so difficult to consume 48 teaspoons of sugar daily. In the following chapters, I shall show how this increased sugar intake results in (1) an increase in body fat and obesity, (2) dietary deficiencies, (3) a decrease in performance, (4) an increase in hyperactivity and other behavioral problems, and (5) an increase in diseases as diverse as cancer, heart disease, and tooth decay.

Foods that contain too much refined flour

The high consumption of white flour also poses a threat to health, although not quite as great as that caused by refined sugar. This threat is due to the fact that the average person is consuming such a large part of his/her diet in the form of white flour and that most of the valuable nutrition has been taken out of this food. In the process of making white flour, the bran and the germ, which contain most of the vitamin and mineral value of the wheat are removed, leaving behind a starchy material which is subsequently ground up into flour. (This same starchy material is also used for the manufacture of farina, wheatena, and cream of wheat, products which share the general poor nutritional characteristics of white flour.)

Loss of Vitamins due to Refining

FOOD	Vitamin						
	Vit. B1	Vit. B2	Vit. B3	Vit. B5	Vit. B6	Vit. Bc	Vit. E
Whole Wheat Flour	1.10˙	0.21	0.68	0.60	0.47	0.41	0.24
White Wheat Flour	0.13	0.10	0.14	0.23	0.07	0.15	0.01
Reduction Due To Refining	**88%**	**54%**	**80%**	**62%**	**84%**	**63%**	**96%**
Wheat Germ	3.69	1.10	0.61	1.10	1.15	2.26	13.8
Wheat Bran	2.25	0.97	5.19	2.48	1.75	3.02	1.45

Loss of Minerals due to Refining

FOOD	Mineral						
	Calcium	Iron	Magnesium	Phosphorus	Potassium	Zinc	Copper
Whole Wheat Flour	0.1˙	0.55	0.85	0.93	0.3	0.05	0.6
White Wheat Flour	0.04	0.13	0.17	0.21	0.07	0.01	0.21
Reduction Due To Refining	**64%**	**76%**	**80%**	**78%**	**77%**	**73%**	**65%**
Wheat Germ	0.17	1.44	2.31	2.57	0.61	0.26	1.43
Wheat Bran	0.47	3.89	5.75	4.99	1.4	0.31	3

*RDAs per 1000 calories

In the preceding tables, data for the Vitamin B1, B2, and B3 values were obtained from the U.S. Department of Agriculture's Computerized "Nutrient Data Base for Standard Reference, Release 5, Full Version". Data for the Vitamin B5, B6, and Bc values were obtained from the "Nutrition Almanac". Data for the Vitamin E values were obtained from Bowes and Church's "Food Values of Portions Commonly Used". Vitamin B1 is thiamine, Vitamin B2 is riboflavin, Vitamin B3 is niacin, Vitamin B5 is pantothenic acid, Vitamin B6 is pyridoxine, Vitamin Bc is folic acid, and Vitamin E is α-tocopherol.

Data for the calcium, iron, potassium, and phosphorus values were obtained from the U.S. Department of Agriculture's Computerized "Nutrient Data Base for Standard Reference, Release 5, Full Version". Data for the magnesium, zinc and copper values were obtained from the "Nutrition Almanac".

The bran and germ, which are rich in vitamins and minerals are fed to animals, because there is money in "healthy" animals. The remaining white flour is sold to us in the form of a variety of junk food products (listed in the above table) which are embalmed with a host of artificial additives and lined up on supermarket shelves where they lie in state waiting for some unsuspecting soul to pick them up.

And do they spoil? No.

Why not? Because any bug or worm that would ever get into these products would die of malnutrition.

The same nutritional losses that occur in the production of white flour also occur when whole wheat is refined into farina, wheatena, or cream of wheat, when brown rice is refined into white rice, when corn is degerminated to make cornmeal or grits, or when any whole grain is stripped of its germ and bran.

After depleting our food of hundreds of nutrients necessary for good health, the food manufacturers tell us they enrich our foods by replenishing four nutrients: vitamin B1, vitamin B2, vitamin B3, and iron. As Joe Nichols, a founder of Natural Food Associates, often said, that is like having some thief take hundreds of dollars out of your pockets, give you four dollars in return, and then tell you that he has enriched you.

Foods that contain trash fats

Without question, trash fat foods like margarine, vegetable shortenings, hydrogenated oils, or partially hydrogenated oils, as well as foods containing them should be avoided. In the manufacture of these products, vegetable oils are hydrogenated, a process which destroys essential polyunsaturated fats, such as linoleic acid and linolenic acid, to produce trash fats (including "trans fatty acids") which your body was never meant to handle. Trash fats gunk up your body's ability to properly utilize beneficial fats and have been linked to cancer and heart disease.

	Polyunsaturated Fats[1]	Vitamin E
Soybean Oil	61%	11
Hydrogenated Soybean Oil	40%	8
Soft Soybean Oil Margarine	35%	2
Hard Soybean Oil Margarine	30%	2
Soybean Oil Shortening	18%	—

---

[1] percentage of total fatty acids 2milligrams per 100 grams of fat
Data for the polyunsaturated fat values were obtained from the U.S. Department of Agriculture's Computerized "Nutrient Data Base for Standard Reference, Release 5, Full Version". Data for the Vitamin E values were obtained from Bowes and Church's "Food Values of Portions Commonly Used".

In this process, Vitamins A, E, and K, lipoic acid, Coenzyme Q, and many other essential nutrients are also lost or destroyed.

To make margarine palatable to the consumer, chemicals are added to make it taste like butter and coloring is added to make it look like butter. In addition, preservatives such as benzoic acid are added to embalm it.

If you want butter, eat butter. However, when you buy butter, see if it is labeled "sweet cream butter". If it isn't, it is likely that the butter was made from sour cream which was neutralized with lye before it was made into butter. Sweet cream butter is available in two forms, lightly salted or unsalted, either of which can be recommended. Butter made from sour cream and neutralized is far superior to margarine, but will be of a slightly lower quality than sweet cream butter.

If, as you start out on the program, you wish to use fats which contain no cholesterol, use cold-pressed vegetable oils, *not margarine*. Make sure you stay away from all oils that are "hydrogenated" or "partially hydrogenated" as well as any food products containing them. If you are cooking with an oil, it is best to use a more saturated oil such as sesame oil, olive oil, or cold-pressed peanut oil. If you are frying with these oils, try not to overheat your pan.

Foods that contain artificial additives

Eating artificial food additives and plastic foods is like playing Russian roulette. While there is a possibility that you can get away using some of them some of the time, one bad episode can take its toll in health and life. Continual use of these products will increase the probability that you will suffer from the adverse effects. Like Russian roulette, you can play the game once, twice, three times . . . but the more you play, the greater your chances are of losing. Cancer from Red Dye #2, headaches from monosodium glutamate, hyperactivity from numerous other additives . . . Are these the chances you want to take with your life and the lives of your children? The warning has been given. Stay away from the foods listed on the "Foods to Stay Away From" table.

Other foods to stay away from

In addition to the foods listed on this table, it is best to stay away from frozen foods other than those that are frozen fresh or blanched. Stay away from foods that have added salt, sugar, sauces or that are prebreaded or precooked. Stay away

from TV dinners, canned stews, canned beans, pastas which
are made from "refined" and "enriched" wheat (I urge spaghetti addicts to replace their pasta with brown rice and try to
"junk out" on white spaghetti no more than 5 times a year).
Canned tomatos and tomato paste can be used to make sauces
like spaghetti sauce, but stay away from premade sauces since
they invariably contain a corn sweetener and other junk. Stay
away from canned fruits and apple sauce with sugar added.
Stay away from dry milk, condensed milk, and artificial
creams and whip creams. In short, stay away from any food
that does not fit within one of the categories of the recommended list of foods.

Coffee, regular tea (tea of thea), and cocoa (chocolate) contain
the stimulants caffeine, theobromine and theophylline, as
well as dangerously high levels of tannins. These items are
drugs, not foods. If drugs are to be used at all, their administration should be short-term and they should be given only
during serious health crises. The common routine usage of
coffee, tea, and cocoa as stimulants is by no means short-
term. It upsets the normal biochemical processes of the cen-
tral nervous system. Normal sleep patterns are disturbed.
Like any other drug that is abused, coffee, tea, and cocoa are
addictive. The tannins that they contain have been associated
with liver and kidney damage. It has been estimated that the
total intake of tannins from coffee, tea, and cocoa for some
drinkers is above the level that would be expected to cause an
effect. With the exception that coffee has relatively high vitamin B3 levels, these items are virtually devoid of any food
value. Coffee, tea and cocoa, as well as foods containing them,
should be avoided.

Regular tea, such as Lipton or Salada, is made from the
evergreen shrub, Camellia sinensis. In contrast, "herbal"
teas, which have traditionally been used for their medicinal
properties, are made from a variety of different herbs. If you
are drinking herbal teas for medicinal purposes, don't drink
them regularly as if they were a food; even herbalists advise
that continual drinking of medicinal teas results in the reduc-

tion of their medicinal properties. If you are drinking them for their nutritional value, remember that steeping herbs in near boiling water will result in a loss of some vitamin value. Along with coffee substitutes such as Postum, Caffix, and others, herbal teas can at least serve the function of providing a substitute for coffee, regular tea, or cocoa for those who might otherwise find them more difficult to get off of.

In any event, stay away from decaffeinated coffee products. The decaffeinating agents used are often a greater health hazard than the caffeine they remove.

For old times sake

Take one more visit down the aisles of the junk food section of your supermarket. Go to the ready-to-eat cereals section. This wasteland of trash, courtesy of General Mills, Nabisco, Ralston Purina, Kellogg's, Post, Quaker Oats, is a monument to the tragedy of the damage which we have helped these companies inflict upon our children and ourselves. Read the labels on some of these cereals:

*** Count Chocula: oat flour, sugar, marbits (sugar, corn starch, dextrose, cocoa, wheat starch, calcium carbonate, trisodium phosphate, artificial flavor), waxy-wax (refined wax, chewing gum base, soy lecithin, artificial color).

*** Apple Jacks: sugar, corn syrup, wheat and nut flour, dried apples, apple juice concentrate, cinnamon, artificial color, vitamins.

*** PacMan Cereal: degerminated corn meal, marbits (sugar, corn starch, dextrose, cocoa, wheat starch, calcium carbonate, trisodium phosphate, artificial flavor), color bubbles (dextrose, sugar, gum base, artificial colors and flavors, confectioner's glaze, BHT).

*** Post Fruity Pebbles: rice, sugar, hydrogenated coconut oil, corn syrup, salt, artificial flavor, vitamins added.

Reading it may be funny. But eating it and feeding it is not.

Physical activity is the spark

Even if you are very careful with what you eat, only by being
physically active can you put the good food you eat to proper
use. For example, as you start the Basic Exercise Program,
you will stimulate your body to produce more hemoglobin, you
will stimulate muscle growth, you will stimulate bone cells to
break down old bone tissue and build new bone tissue, you will
stimulate metabolic and detoxification processes generally,
etc., etc. . . . It is only then that the protein, the iron, the
calcium, and the many other essential factors in food can be
drawn into the areas where they can do the most good.

In the complete absence of physical stress, the degenerative
effects can be seen almost immediately. For example, when
astronauts spend time out in space under weightless conditions, they experience a loss of bone mass and muscle tone, as
well as a deterioration of other vital functions.

In nature (back on earth), gravity provides you nourishment
in the form of force. Finding gravity is not the problem. The
problem is knowing how to equip yourself with the proper
tools to take full advantage of the beneficial effects of gravity
and making up your mind that you are going to set aside at
least 3-4 hours a week and take the time to do something for
your body — the most important physical thing you own.

How to get your exercise paraphernalia

You can purchase your workout clothes at any clothing store
or sporting goods store. Your workout clothes should be loose
fitting or very stretchy. For workouts I wear a medium to
heavy weight T-shirt, a pair of shorts with an expandable
waistband, and a pair of athletic sox, all made of 100% cotton.
For undergarments, cotton briefs are adequate. Men may
prefer wearing an athletic supporter and women may consider

wearing an athletic bra. For outergarments, I recommend a loose-fitting sweat shirt and sweat pants, also of 100% cotton.

Ideally, if you are a beginner, it doesn't pay to buy your own workout equipment. It is best to join a health club near you so that you can make the most of your time. In general, the memberships will run from about 20 to 40 dollars per month for an individual membership, with substantial discounts for family memberships. (Some extremely plush facilities will run higher.) If you do a fair amount of traveling, you might be interested in joining a club that allows you to use other health facilities throughout the U.S. Before deciding on a health club, take this book with you and show them the workout schedules. Get an assurance from them, in writing, that they have facilities which are adequate to handle the workout schedules outlined in this book. Find out whether there are capable people on the staff who are available to take you through the workout schedule and assist you in developing proper form. A properly chosen health club will be worth far more than its weight in gold.

After working out for six months or a year, you might consider equipping your own workout facility. Similarly, those who cannot find a health club that is convenient for them might consider getting their own workout facility. [See Appendix]

In selecting running shoes and a bicycle, don't try to pinch pennies. For shoes, go to a sporting goods store, a triathlete shop, or an athletic shoe store and take the time to get your shoes professionally fit. To purchase a bicycle, go to a bicycle shop and have a bicycle professionally fitted to you. A good bicycle will cost you in the range of $300 to $500. While cycling is a pleasant and beneficial way to exercise, **under no circumstances should you delay going on or continuing with the program because you can't afford to purchase a good bicycle.** Specialty clothing is available for running and bicycling. I advise sticking with natural fabrics, especially cotton, wherever possible.

Chapter 6

Balancing Your Needs

Y our body is composed of a framework of bones (your skeleton). These bones form an intricate system of levers which are held together by strong elastic structures called ligaments. Muscles, which are attached to bones by tendons and are surrounded by tendinous membranes called fascia, provide the energy to move your skeletal structure. Muscles do this because they have the ability to contract. For example, when you "make a muscle" with your arm, your biceps contracts and becomes thicker. In this process, your fist is drawn towards your shoulder. As you straighten out your arm, your biceps relaxes and a muscle connected to the same bones on the opposite side (called the triceps) contracts to provide you the energy to extend your arm to its original position. These muscles, not surprisingly, are called skeletal muscles (e.g. the heart, which is a muscle, is not a skeletal muscle). Your bones move about joints which are lined with a smooth substance called cartilage.

Your bones aren't stones. They are composed of living cells called osteoclasts, which break down old bone tissue, and other cells called osteoblasts, which build up new bone tissue. Exercise stimulates the activity of osteoclasts to break down old bone tissue; it also stimulates osteoblasts to synthesize and release (to the outside of the cell) a protein called collagen. When released, this collagen becomes mineralized to form new hard bone tissue. While exercise is required to keep the process going, periods of rest and sleep are also necessary to allow the body to concentrate on bone building. This bone rejuvenation also requires a supply of protein, calcium, vitamin C, and other nutrients to provide the building materials. Thus, if you fail to exercise, rest, or eat the foods necessary to provide these nutrients, bone rejuvenation will be impaired and bones will begin to deteriorate.

Similarly, exercise, proper nutrition, and rest stimulate the rejuvenation and strengthening of tendons, ligaments, and cartilage. Like the osteoblasts of bone tissue, tendons, ligaments, and cartilage have collagen-forming cells called fibroblasts (in tendons and ligaments) and chondroblasts (in cartilage). The collagen produced by these tissues is subtly different from the collagen produced in bone and, as a result, is not calcified. This uncalcified collagen has the resilience and elasticity required for the functions of ligaments, tendons, and cartilage. Continual exposure to poisons in the environment, such as fluoride, interferes with these subtle differences, and as a result, collagen in bone tissue which should be calcified is not (resulting in a disease called osteomalacia) — and collagen in ligaments, tendons, and cartilage, which should not be calcified, is (resulting in torn muscles, ligaments, and tendons as well as osteoarthritis).

Bones, muscles, tendons, and all of the other tissues of the body are supplied with nutrients through the blood, which the heart pumps to these tissues through blood vessels called arteries and capillaries. The blood receives these nutrients primarily through the lungs, stomach, and intestines. With the help of ducts in the body which collect fluid (lymph) and deposit it into the blood, blood also removes waste products from these tissues. Various other organs, such as the liver, the kidney, the spleen, the thymus, the bone marrow, and the lungs remove waste products from the blood by detoxifying them and eliminating them from the body.

Oxygen is the most important nutrient — and increasing your ability to deliver it throughout the body and utilize it is a major factor in improving your performance.

By exercising, you increase your blood's ability to carry oxygen to the tissues. Here is how it works. You start an exercise and your heart rate and breathing rate automatically begin to pick up. You get to the point where you can no longer increase either your breathing rate or your heart rate and yet your body is still crying for more oxygen. As a result, you begin to slow down, even if you push yourself.

When you are done with the exercise, your body realizes that you may put it through another similar ordeal. Not wanting to go through this again, your body prepares itself by building more capillaries and increasing blood supply to the muscles. It also increases the amount of hemoglobin (the protein that carries most of the oxygen from the lungs to the muscles) in blood as well as the number of mitochondria (little particles in the cell which are responsible for using oxygen to burn food and produce energy) and the amount of myoglobin (the protein that carries oxygen from the cell surface to the mitochondria) in muscles. These adaptations require protein, iron, riboflavin, and other nutrients to provide the building materials. Continual exposure to poisons in the environment, such as carbon monoxide (which ties up hemoglobin and prevents it from carrying oxygen), interferes with your ability to increase the supply of oxygen to your body.

In muscle (including heart), exercise also stimulates other physiological and biochemical changes which result in greater strength, speed, and endurance. As you exercise, your muscles increase in size. Your body becomes more efficient, that is, more energy from the food your body burns is used to perform the activity you are engaged in and less is wasted as heat. [During the first few weeks of the program, those of you who have not been on an exercise program recently may feel a burning sensation in your muscles while exercising. This will go away as your body starts to resurrect itself.]

In other tissues (such as the liver, kidney, spleen, thymus, bone marrow, and lungs), the physiological and biochemical changes that are induced by exercise and rest supported by a proper diet improves the strength of your immune system as well as your body's ability to detoxify its waste products and eliminate them from the body. These changes also result in a cleaner and more efficient digestive tract.

The brain coordinates the functions of the body by sending out a network of nerves which provide a sensory system for receiving signals from other parts of the body and a control mechanism for directing the movement of muscles. The brain also directs overall body metabolism by the secretion of hormones into the blood and continually monitors the blood for hormones and other substances to help it determine whether changes in its instructions to the body are necessary.

Exercise helps provide a better supply of more oxygenated blood to the brain, improving the brain's ability to perform its functions. Exercise also trains the brain to more effectively coordinate muscular activity. For example, if you are lifting a heavy weight, it is necessary for you to get your muscle cells to "fire off" at the same time in order to lift the weight. If the firing off occurs haphazardly or in some random fashion, you may not be able to lift the weight. The training effect of lifting heavier weights allows your brain to make adjustments that result in better performance on subsequent workouts.

When you begin an exercise, your brain (without your conscious knowledge) calculates the amount of energy needed, the time for which it is needed, and the type of fuel to burn during the exercise period. Exercise trains your brain to make these determinations more accurately. Based on these determinations, commands from the brain are carried to the tissues in the form of nerve impulses and hormonal secretions. For example, if your brain senses that you need to act quickly, it signals the release of the hormone adrenalin which increases the metabolism of glycogen. This provides a quick burst of energy, which can be maintained for only a short amount of time. If your brain senses that you are going to run a marathon (26-mile) race, it signals the release of a hormone called the somatotrophic hormone, which increases the metabolism of fats and possibly a small amount of protein, providing for the production of energy over an extended period of time. By combining these and many other factors, the brain tries to provide you with the best fuel mixture for optimal performance.

In addition to stimulating the proper secretion of metabolic hormones, exercise (supported with periods of rest, nutritional support, and avoidance of harmful drugs or other environmental poisons) stimulates the secretion of hormones responsible for optimal growth, development, and sexual drive.

In order to receive messages and transmit commands, the brain requires a whole slew of nutrients including protein, nucleic acids, choline, sodium, potassium, and many, many others. In order to utilize glycogen, fats, or proteins as fuels, the cells in the body also need nutrients, including nucleic acids, phosphorus, niacin, carnitine, lipoic acid, thiamin, pantothenic acid, coenzyme Q, and many, many others.

So long as you stick with the recommended list of foods, your brain will know and direct you to eat the types of foods you need to keep your body functioning properly. For most of you, who have strayed from these foods, tables will be provided to help get you back on the right track.

Your brain has quite a job to do! That is why a positive mental attitude is so important. If you convince yourself you can do something, your brain will readjust itself to help make it happen. If you take a negative attitude, things that you should have been able to accomplish become impossible. If you allow your mind to become sloppy, accidents result. In the High Performance Health Program, mental attitude is the key. Diligently following the program and believing in it, your brain will make your body adjust as you get it off of cigarets, coffee, drugs, junk foods, and other harmful substances in your environment and as you get it on a program rich in good nutrition and physical activity.

Keeping your mind uncluttered helps your brain devote more time to take care of its physical responsibilities. This means that rather than worrying about something, you should do something about it. If, after trying, you find you can't do anything about it, get it out of your mind. Easy to say, isn't it? But if you don't, the negative thoughts and resentments that your brain has to continually and unnecessarily deal with will have a negative effect on your health. A positive mental attitude — based upon realistically facing up to problems, dealing with them as effectively as you can, and feeling satisfied when you know that you've done all you can — will have an extremely positive effect on your health.

Your brain has quite a job to do! That's why it shuts down most of its functions and puts you to sleep for 7-9 hours each day (if you let it). While the rest of your body is relaxing, repairing, and rejuvenating itself, the brain finds the time to sort through old trash that it would like to get rid of and makes you conscious of it in dreams or upon waking the following morning. It also reorders the important items for you to consider to allow you to take a fresh look at them the following morning when you wake up.

In short, the benefits of the High Performance Health Program include the following:

- strengthening and rejuvenation of ligaments, tendons, joints and bones.
- increasing muscle strength, speed, and endurance.
- improving the capacity and health of your heart.
- improving blood circulation.
- improving the oxygen capacity and health of your blood.
- improving the capacity and health of your lungs.
- improving the oxygen capacity and health of every cell in your body.
- strengthening the immune system.
- improving the detoxification and excretory functions.

- stimulating mental function.
- stimulating appropriate hormone secretion, metabolism, and sexual drive.
- stimulating appropriate appetite.
- increasing muscle mass.
- decreasing body fat.
- looking good.
- feeling good.

Balancing the foods you eat

"One thing I have learned in a long life: that all science, measured against reality, is primitive and childlike."
Albert Einstein

The program is simple. Despite the large number of different good foods that are available, your body, sparked on by physical activity, will lead you to balance the foods you eat to provide the nutrients your body needs. In this chapter, I have provided lists of foods high in various nutrients. By following the general guidelines accompanying these lists and by choosing foods from these lists, you can use these lists as "training wheels" until you clean up your body and gain more confidence in its abilities. Performance tests, which will be described in a later chapter, will give you an objective tool to fine tune your diet.

This program is a revolutionary departure from other programs. It works because it takes into consideration the fact that science as we now know it is not now nor will it ever be in a position to unravel the complexities of isolating every single nutrient, let alone determine the functions of each and understand their interrelationships for every situation that arises at each stage in our development. Yet this program takes the best that science has to offer and uses it for your advantage. The arrogance of other programs "based on science" has virtually neglected the built-in abilities of the human brain to put together all this information and come out with a correct answer in a matter of seconds. They have also failed to understand the limitations of current scientific knowledge.

For example, of the hundreds of thousands of different nutrients that naturally occur in foods, less than 50 are currently recognized as "essential". The true number of "essential" nutrients, some of which will still be unknown to us 1000 years from now, is far higher.

Nutrients Currently Recognized as Essential

Vitamin A	Vitamin E	Vitamin K	Linoleic Acid
Tryptophan	Threonine	Lysine	Methionine
Valine	Leucine	Isoleucine	Phenylalanine
Histidine	Vitamin C	Thiamine	Riboflavin
Pantothenate	Pyridoxine	Vitamin B12	Folic acid
Biotin	Water	Calcium	Potassium
Sodium	Chlorine	Phosphorus	Magnesium
Iron	Copper	Manganese	Selenium
Zinc	Iodine		

Cobalt (in vitamin B12)
Chromium (in glucose tolerance factor)
Carbon (in proteins, fats, carbohydrates, and nucleic acids)
Hydrogen (in proteins, fats, carbohydrates, and nucleic acids)
Oxygen (in air, proteins, fats, carbohydrates, and nucleic acids)
Nitrogen (in proteins and nucleic acids)
Sulfur (in proteins and carbohydrates)

Niacin (vitamin B3) is not necessary if there is enough tryptophan (from protein) in the diet. Cholecalciferol, erroneously called vitamin D, is a hormone made in the skin from cholesterol. In order to synthesize this hormone, the skin requires sunlight. Fluoride, a poison used to kill cockroaches, rats, and silverfish, has been referred to as an essential nutrient for political reasons, despite the fact that a fluoride deficiency has never been found in man or animal.

Other Nutrients Essential or Important to Human Life

Stigmasterol	Hematin	Nucleic Acids	Pteridines
Eicosapentanoic Acid	Glutathione	Nitrilosides	Carnitine
Para-aminobenzoic Acid	Pangamic Acid	Bioflavinoids	Proteins
Bifidus Factor	Carotenoids	Choline	Inositol
Docosapentanoic Acid	Coenzyme Q	Lipoic Acid	Peptides

The usefulness of knowing where to find the *known* essential nutrients is that from this knowledge, we can get an indication of where to find the far greater number of *unknown* essential nutrients and other important nutrients in the foods we eat. Also, avoiding foods in which the known essential nutrients have been destroyed by food preparation techniques will help us avoid foods in which the unknown essential nutrients and other important nutrients have been lost or destroyed.

Fats

From natural foods, you probably receive over 100,000 different fats in your diet. Fats provide a major source of energy in the body. However, fats also provide a number of very important factors which are necessary for the proper functioning of your body including your body's ability to burn up food and use it for energy. Some of these chemicals include vitamins A, E, and K, Coenzyme Q, lecithin, lipoic acid, linoleic acid, linolenic acid, arachadonic acid, eicosapentanoic acid, and docosahexanoic acid.

Excluding *particular* fats from your diet can cause problems. For example, it has been my observation that many female athletes whose body fat falls below 12% experience a loss of their normal monthly cycle when they try to keep a fat called cholesterol out of their diet. Because their body stores of fat are so low and because they burn up foods so rapidly in order to maintain their high activity levels, they may lack enough cholesterol to produce the progesterone and estrogen (their estrogen levels are only one-third that of female athletes with a regular cycle) necessary to maintain estrus and, when this happens, their periods stop. If they are on a reasonably high cholesterol diet, I have found that they are able to maintain their normal monthly cycles even at body fat levels as low as 6%.

For those of you who might welcome the termination of your periods, I should remind you that it is an indication that your health has reached a low level. Estrus is something you can do without temporarily; however, the loss of estrus may be the last warning signal you have that your body is going to economize with cholesterol usage in other more critical places (such as the maintenence of cell walls necessary for proper nerve conduction).

Male athletes are less fortunate in that they do not have such an obvious warning system. It is possible that a low body fat coupled with an extreme low-cholesterol diet could produce a fall-off in testosterone that would adversely affect their development and physical performance (since testosterone in the body helps to increase muscle mass and decrease body fat) as well as their sexual performance. This fall-off in testosterone might also be reflected in a drop-off in sperm count.

The use of anabolic steroid drugs such as testosterone and its synthetic derivatives by some of these athletes is the ultimate mistake. While temporarily allowing physical development to proceed, these drugs suppress testosterone synthesis by the body, resulting in a decrease in the function and size of the testes over time. When anabolic steroid drug use is discontinued, the body's ability to again produce testosterone is often reduced to the point that muscle mass is lost and body fat begins to increase. By this time, serious decreases in sperm counts can be expected.

To avoid these problems, you must rely on a good diet **and** a good exercise program. Extremely low fat diets should be avoided. In addition, the quality of the fats consumed should be high and the sources of the fats consumed should be varied.

Natural unprocessed foods provide the best source of fat. Raw nuts, seeds, and avocados are excellent sources of quality fats, but it must be remembered that 75-90% of the caloric value of these foods is present as fat, so moderation in their consumption should be exercised. The following table provides a list of other natural foods and the percentage of calories that is present as fat.

Fat Content of Various Food Groups

Food Group	Fat Content
Untrimmed Meat	60-85%
Eggs and Cheeses	60-80%
Meat (from fatty fish such as mackerel and trout)	50-60%
Whole "cow's" milk	50%
Trimmed Meat	40-60%
Organs (heart, liver, and kidney)	25-50%
Meat (from other fish)	5-30%
Grains, Beans, Vegetables, and Fruits	0-15%

Values given as percent of the total caloric value of the food. As used in this book, "meat" refers to the skeletal muscles of animals that are used as food.

Since the types of fat derived from each of these sources differ, it is wise to get as much variety in your diet as possible, keeping a close watch to make sure that your body can tolerate each of the foods in your diet. (Foods which bring on allergic reactions, produce excess mucus, result in irregular heart beats, or in any other way interfere with your performance should be avoided.)

Recently fish, in particular oily fish and fish oils, have become a fad because they contain a neglected group of fats, referred to as omega fatty acids (such as eicosapentanoic acid and docosahexanoic acid). People with a diet rich in these foods appear to have a lower heart disease rate. Whether or not these fats are responsible for "healthier" hearts, one thing is clear — you can't wait until next year to find out which of the other 500,000 or so nutrients that our food provides is "discovered" as the wonder nutrient of the year. By sticking with the foods on the recommended list, you will already be getting these nutrients. [By the way, the reason that fish have such high levels of these fats is that their food chain includes plants that have even higher levels of them. Omega fatty acids have been found in algae, mosses, and ferns and most recently in green leafy vegetables, so there is no reason for strict vegetarians to worry about not having marine fish oils in their diet.]

Sticking exclusively with the above foods as a source of fat would be best for your health. However, some types of food preparation rely upon using fats and oils that have been fractionated from the above foods in the form of tallow, lard, butter, or oil and people generally insist on eating foods prepared in this manner.

When oil is pressed from vegetable sources (such as olives, sesame seeds, peanuts, corn, cottonseeds, and soybeans), it can be (1) "cold pressed" or (2) extracted with chemicals (hexane) and refined (fractionated further, deodorized, bleached, etc.).

It is advisable to stay away from oils that are not cold pressed since oils which are not cold pressed lose a good portion of their vitamin A and vitamin E and other naturally occurring fats during processing. For example, if your oil is not cold-pressed, a group of fats called phospholipids, which include lecithin, are removed. It is this group of fats that is necessary for the proper mobilization and metabolism of other fats in the body. In addition, some chemical alteration of the fats in non-cold pressed oils occurs during processing, the effects of which could result in an alteration in fat metabolism, and minute amounts of hexane can be found in these oils.

Olive oil and sesame oil are usually cold-pressed. When buying other oils, make sure that they are labeled "cold pressed". Some oils like cottonseed oil (cottonseeds were probably never intended for human consumption) are not available in cold-pressed form because they contain natural toxic chemicals (such as gossypol) which must be removed. Cold-pressed soybean oil, in my opinion, tastes horrible, but then again, it is also my opinion that soybeans and soybean products were probably never meant for human consumption anyway (even farm animals which get out into a soybean field can die from eating soybeans). There is a large selection of cold-pressed oils that are available at health food stores and co-ops, including olive, sesame, peanut, corn, safflower, sunflower, almond, coconut, etc. Some of these oils are slowly finding there way into supermarkets.

Some of the chemically processed, highly refined oils are also hydrogenated or partially hydrogenated. As I pointed out in Chapter 5, hydrogenated fats such as margarine, vegetable shortenings, hydrogenated oils, or partially hydrogenated oils, as well as foods containing them should be avoided. During the hydrogenation process, essential polyunsaturated fats, such as linoleic acid and linolenic acid, are destroyed to produce trash fats (including "trans fatty acids") which your body was never meant to handle. Trash fats gunk up your body's ability to properly utilize beneficial fats and have been linked to cancer and heart disease.

If that isn't enough, some of these highly refined oils and hydrogenated oils contain BHA, BHT, benzoic acid, and other chemicals which are used as embalming agents. To make margarine palatable to the consumer, chemicals are added to make it taste like butter and coloring is added to make it look like butter.

If you are cooking with a fat, it is best to use butter or a more saturated oil such as sesame oil, olive oil, or cold-pressed peanut oil. If you are frying with these oils, try not to overheat your pan. The other more unsaturated cold-pressed oils should *not* be used for cooking because they have a greater tendency to break down to form toxic substances when heated. However, you may use them for salad dressings, mayonnaises, or other non-heated food products. When buying the more unsaturated oils, taste them to see if they are rancid. If they are, return them. If they pass the taste test, store them in a cold, dark place until you use them up.

During the separation of milk to produce the cream to make butter, phospholipids, such as lecithin, are lost (they remain in the skim milk). However, butter is very rich in certain fats (known as "short-chain fatty acids") which are not readily found in other foods. These fats exist in other dairy products, such as milk and cheese as well. However, considering that butter is the best tolerated dairy product, its inclusion in your diet might be worthwhile as a source of these rare fats.

Other than providing the same energy and fats that your own body stores of fat already provide you with, tallow and lard, while they are the most stable natural fats to cook with, have little if any added nutritional value. The composition of these fats can vary based on what the animal eats. In contrast, the type of fat found in the fruits and grains used to make vegetable oil is more constant because each of these foods derives its fats only from what its parent plant synthesizes and from what its characteristic needs are. Fat from eggs and dairy products, since both are designed to provide for food for a future generation, also tends to have a more predictable composition, although even they can vary as is evidenced by the higher carotene content that can be noticed, e.g. in the bright orange yolks of range fed chickens or in the yellower color of cream of range fed cows.

You should avoid fried foods whenever you eat out. You never know what they use to fry foods in, but more often than not, it is some chemically extracted, synthetically hydrogenated, chemically embalmed fat that is not only of low quality, but also contains synthetic components that your body can't handle. For the same reason, it is wise to avoid salad oils and salad dressings while eating out. (If you wish to have a salad oil when eating out, you might consider putting a 4-ounce bottle of olive oil in your pocket or pocketbook and use it along with the vinegar or the lemon juice of lemon wedges which are invariably available at all but the scummiest of restaurants.) The same goes for foods you buy at the supermarket. You are much better off not buying oil-containing foods.

For example, 60% of the calories you get from potato chips comes from the fat that they were cooked in. In most cases, this tremendous amount of fat is hydrogenated junk fat. This fat is used to fry the potatoes to the point that many of the beneficial nutrients in the potato have been destroyed. When shopping in the supermarket, read your labels and at least stay away from foods such as corn chips, mayonnaises, salad dressings, baked goods, or any other products that use hydrogenated or partially hydrogenated oils. If you are going to use these foods, the best thing to do is to make them yourself or find some company that uses cold-pressed oils to make them with. These products can usually be found at health food stores and food co-ops, but even there, be sure to read your labels.

Even if you make fat-containing foods at home, watch the amount of fat you eat. For example, the amount of fat contained in fried foods is surprisingly high. Forty to fifty percent of the calories you eat in potatoes fried at home comes from the fat you fry them in. Twenty-five to thirty-five percent of the calories you eat in pancakes comes from the fat you fry them in. So use these foods in moderation and try, when cooking, to also prepare foods that are raw, steamed, boiled, baked, roasted, or broiled.

Remember, fats are an important ingredient in your diet and are necessary for the proper functioning of your body. So eat the highest quality fats that you can and avoid the trash fat foods. This will become one of the foundation stones of improving your performance and your body shape.

Carbohydrates

From natural foods, you receive a large number of different carbohydrates. Carbohydrates, in the form of complex carbohydrates (such as starch) and simple sugars (such as glucose, fructose, and sucrose), provide a major source of energy for your body. The necessity or importance of the many other carbohydrates or carbohydrate-like substances is, for the most part, unknown. Vitamin C is the only carbohydrate-like substance that is currently regarded as essential. However, others, such as a carbohydrate known as "Bifidus Factor" and a carbohydrate-like substance called inositol, have also been found to be essential or important to human health. Even fiber, which consists of indigestible carbohydrates such as cellulose, is now regarded as beneficial. The key is that by staying with natural foods, you will be receiving all these carbohydrates and others without having to wait for some great scientist to isolate them and determine that they are important in your diet.

Most of the energy-producing (digestible) carbohydrate in the diet that is absorbed into the body is either stored in muscles and liver in the form of glycogen or broken down to a substance called pyruvic acid to yield energy. The production of this energy *requires no oxygen* and is called *anaerobic* glycolysis (glycolysis means sugar breakdown). The pyruvic acid is then either (1) temporarily stored in the form of lactic acid, (2) stored more permanently as fat, or (3) broken down to carbon dioxide and water to yield energy (this process, which *requires oxygen*, releases over 90% of the energy provided by carbohydrates and is called *aerobic* glycolysis). About 99% (300-400 grams) of the carbohydrate in your body is stored as glycogen. Very little remains in the blood as sugar (only about 4 grams or one-seventh of an ounce).

During intensive short-term exercises, most of the energy used comes from from anaerobic breakdown of carbohydrate. On slightly longer-term exercises, the majority of energy comes from the aerobic breakdown of carbohydrate. On long-term exercises, fat becomes the predominant fuel used.

Energy Source During Maximal Exercise For Various Times

| Exercise Time | Energy Source | | |
	Carbohydrate Anaerobic (Calories)	Carbohydrate Aerobic Equivalents (Calories)	Net Fat Aerobic (Calories)
10 seconds	20	4	0
1 minute	30	20	0
2 minutes	30	45	0
5 minutes	30	120	0
10 minutes	25	245	0
30 minutes	20	240	435
60 minutes	15	180	1020

Based on data presented by Gollnick and Hermanson, 1973 and the generally recognized assumption that aerobic metabolism of glucose from glycogen generates 12 times more energy than its anaerobic metabolism.

Fat actually is being burned off in the 10-second to 10-minute exercises. However anaerobic carbohydrate breakdown produces substances which must subsequently be burned off later in place of the fat that would normally have been burned off. This results in a net fat burnoff of zero. Only after working out continuously for 15 minutes or more do you seriously *begin* to start burning off fat.

The table also shows that by setting your mind to doing a longer workout, less carbohydrate and more fat is utilized. Notice, for example, how by exercising maximally for one hour, less carbohydrate is used anaerobically than during a maximal 10 second exercise.

The glycogen content in active people (about one pound) is substantially higher than that of inactive people. This pound of glycogen is enough to provide a total of approximately 1800 calories; however, the body of an active person will start burning fat after the first quarter ounce of glycogen has been used up. An active person (e.g. a 120 pound woman with a body fat of 12% or a 180 pound man with a body fat of 8%) will have a total body fat of 14-15 pounds which can provide a total of approximately 60,000 calories of energy. Needless to say, body fat can provide a lot more energy than stored carbohydrates.

In inactive people, body fats of 30-50% yielding 50-100 pounds of body fat can provide up to 400,000 calories of energy. This excess fat hinders performance and is as useful and as attractive as an extra 200-gallon tank of gas strapped to the roof of a Volkswagen. This excess fat must be burned off before you can get into decent shape. However, in order to burn off fat, longer endurance-type workouts are necessary.

Despite the fact that inactive people have less carbohydrate (stored as glycogen) in their bodies, they rely more heavily on carbohydrates for their fuel source. This is because their blood is poorly oxygenated and because the cells in their body are poor in the myoglobin and mitochondria necessary to burn fat. They derive shots of energy from the anaerobic breakdown of carbohydrate to pyruvic acid, which they temporarily store as lactic acid and then slowly turn into either fat (which contributes to obesity and high cholesterol) or carbon dioxide and water (for additional energy). Active people save their glycogen supplies and use the larger supplies of stored fat as an energy source when they are at rest. The following table illustrates this difference between active and inactive people.

Energy Source Used by Heart Muscle of Active and Inactive People at Rest, During a Workout, and During Recovery

Activity Level	Energy Source		
	Fat Aerobic (Calories)	Carbohydrate Aerobic (Calories)	Carbohydrate Anaerobic (Calories)
At Rest			
Active People	53%	20%	27%
Inactive People	38%	31%	31%
After 12-Minute Workout			
Active People	33%	45%	22%
Inactive People	25%	60%	15%
After 15-Minute Recovery			
Active People	48%	33%	19%
Inactive People	33%	42%	25%

* Data from *The Applied Exercise Physiology*, Lea & Febinger, 1982, P. 158

In short, even though they generally carry around less weight, active people have more available energy, have more muscle power, and perform better than inactive people.

Because inactive people rely more on carbohydrate as a fuel source, they tend to eat more carbohydrate - especially in the form of sugar. Eating large amounts of sugar, which is absorbed more rapidly than starches, provides them with a quick high. However, this is often followed by an over-response of insulin which leads to low blood sugar levels, which in turn brings on headaches or a feeling of fatigue. Inactivity coupled to a high consumption of sugar creates an ideal set of conditions for body deterioration and an excellent environment for cancer cell growth.

Eating digestible complex carbohydrates (such as starch), which consist of a long chains of sugars tied together, gives you a greater feeling of fullness and satisfaction, since complex carbohydrates are broken down slowly to provide a more steady supply of sugar to the bloodstream. Over-responses of insulin and some of the other undesirable effects of high sugar eating are less likely to occur when you eat these complex carbohydrates.

Fruits, vegetables, beans, and grains are rich in carbohydrates. Per calorie eaten, nuts and seeds have a much lower carbohydrate content. The following table provides a list of the percentage of calories in each of these food groups that is present as carbohydrate.

Carbohydrate Content of Various Food Groups

Food	Carbohydrate Content
Fruits	90-100%
Vegetables	60-90%
Grains	65-75%
Beans	55-65%
Nuts and Seeds	5-20%

Values given as percent of the total caloric value of the food.

Vegetables, beans, nuts, grains, and seeds contain much less sugar but a greater percentage of digestible complex carbohydrate than fruit. The following table lists the percentages of carbohydrates which are present as sugar, fiber, and as digestible complex carbohydrates, such as starch.

Types of Carbohydrate in Various Food Groups

Food Group	Percent as Sugar	Percent as Fiber	Percent as Digestible Complex Carbohydrate
Grains	.5-2%	10%	90%
Beans	8-16%	20%	64-72%
Nuts & Seeds	10-30%	20%	50-70%
Vegetables	10-80%	10-30%	0-80%
Fruits	40-80%	10-30%	0-40%

Grains and beans have the highest content of complex carbohydrates. The complex carbohydrate content of grains and beans is so high (as can be seen from the following two tables) that it is virtually impossible to eat them without soaking or milling them. Soaked grains and beans can then be cooked or sprouted. Milled grains can be cooked for cereal (e.g. cracked wheat, oatmeal, or cereal) or incorporated into baked goods. Simple recipes for doing this are given in the following chapter

Types of Carbohydrate in Various Grains

Grains (uncooked)	Total Carbohydrate*	Percent as Sugar	Percent as Fiber (estimated)	Percent as Digestible Complex Carbohydrate
Whole Wheat	72.0	0.6%	10%	89.4%
Brown Rice	77.4	0.4%	10%	89.6%
Oats	67.0	0.6%	10%	89.4%
Popcorn	72.1	1.8%	10%	88.2%
Avg for Grains	72.1	0.8%	10%	89.1%

The data on this table and the following table are derived from the U.S. Department of Agriculture's Computerized "Nutrient Data Base for Standard Reference, Release 5, Full Version", the U.S. Department of Agriculture's Provisional Table on the Sugar Content of Selected Foods (October 1986), and from Bowes and Church's "Food Values of Portions Commonly Used", 1985.
*Grams per 100 grams of food.

Types of Carbohydrate in Various Beans

Dry Beans (uncooked)	Total Carbohydrate*	Percent As Sugar	Percent As Fiber (estimated)	Percent As Digestible Complex Carbohydrate
Pink	64.2	8%	10%	82%
Black Beans	62.4	8%	10%	82%
Small White	62.3	8%	10%	82%
Pinto	63.4	8%	10%	82%
Navy	60.7	8%	10%	82%
Broad	58.3	9%	10%	81%
Gt. Northern Beans	62.4	9%	10%	81%
Kidney	60.0	9%	10%	81%
Lima	63.0	12%	10%	78%
Split Peas	60.4	12%	10%	78%
Chickpeas	60.7	16%	10%	74%
AVG FOR BEANS	61.2	10%	10%	80%

*Grams per 100 grams of food.

Nuts and seeds have a much lower content of complex carbohydrates (due primarily to their high fat content) and therefore they can be eaten raw.

Types of Carbohydrate in Various Nuts and Seeds

Nuts & Seeds (Raw)	Total Carbohydrate*	Percent As Sugar	Percent As Fiber (estimated)	Percent As Digestible Complex Carbohydrate
Pumpkin Seeds	17.8	6%	20%	74%
English Walnuts	18.3	11%	20%	69%
Sesame Seeds	9.4	13%	20%	67%
Sunflower Seeds	18.8	18%	20%	62%
Brazilnuts	12.8	22%	20%	58%
Coconut	15.2	23%	20%	57%
Pecans	18.2	24%	20%	56%
Peanuts	16.2	27%	20%	53%
Pistachio Nuts	24.8	27%	20%	53%
Almonds	20.4	29%	20%	51%
Macadamia Nuts	13.7	48%	20%	32%
AVG FOR NUTS	16.9	22%	20%	50%

The data on this table and the following table are derived from the U.S. Department of Agriculture's Computerized "Nutrient Data Base for Standard Reference, Release 5, Full Version", the U.S. Department of Agriculture's Provisional Table on the Sugar Content of Selected Foods (October 1986), and from Bowes and Church's "Food Values of Portions Commonly Used", 1985.
*Grams per 100 grams of food.

Vegetables and fruits have an even lower content of of complex carbohydrates (due primarily to their high water content) and also can be eaten raw.

Types of Carbohydrate in Various Vegetables

Dry Beans (Uncooked)	Total Carbohydrate*	Percent As Sugar	Percent As Fiber	Percent As Digestible Complex Carbohydrate
Asparagus**	3.7	76%	24%	0%
Brussels Sprouts	7.9	31%	28%	41%
Cabbage	5.4	80%	20%	0%
Carrots	10.1	46%	15%	39%
Corn	19.0	19%	8%	72%
Cucumber	2.9	65%	17%	18%
Eggplant	6.3	53%	24%	23%
Kohlrabi	6.2	63%	18%	19%
Leeks	14.2	24%	8%	67%
Lettuce	2.3	49%	30%	22%
Onion	7.3	77%	11%	13%
Pea	14.5	32%	24%	45%
Pepper Steak	5.3	53%	21%	27%
Spinach**	3.5	14%	86%	0%
Summer Squash	4.4	51%	25%	24%
Sweetpotatoes	24.3	16%	9%	75%
Tomato	4.3	67%	18%	15%
Salsify	18.6	8%		
Dandelion Greens	9.2	13%		
Jerusalem Artichoke	17.4	14%		
Rhubarb	4.5	20%		
Potato	18.0	22%		
Broccoli	5.2	34%		
Okra	7.6	38%		
Cauliflower	4.9	49%		
Fennel Leaves	5.1	51%		
Red Cabbage	6.1	57%		
Radishes	3.6	61%		
Chicory Greens	4.7	66%		
Pumpkin	6.5	68%		
Beets	10.0	87%		
Avg. for Vegtables	8.3	45%		

*Grams per 100 grams of food.
**These values were normalized; otherwise, the last column figure would have been a small negative number.

Types of Carbohydrate in Various Fruits

Fruits (Raw)	Total Carbohydrate*	Percent As Sugar	Percent As Fiber	Percent As Digestible Complex Carbohydrate
Apple	15.3	65%	13%	22%
Apricot	11.1	67%	12%	22%
Banana	23.4	60%	6%	34%
Blackberries	12.8	43%	36%	21%
Cherry	16.6	72%	9%	19%
Currants	15.4	52%	35%	13%
Blueberries	14.1	41%		
Raspberries	11.6	47%		
Pear	15.1	53%		
Peach	11.1	60%		
Plum	13.0	66%		
Tangerine	11.2	67%		
Orange	11.8	70%		
Strawberries	7.0	74%		
Grapes	17.2	79%		
Gooseberries	10.2	83%		
Grapefruit	8.1	84%		
AVG FOR FRUITS	13.2	64%		

The data on this table are derived from the U.S. Department of Agriculture's Computerized "Nutrient Data Base for Standard Reference, Release 5, Full Version", the U.S. Department of Agriculture's Provisional Table on the Sugar Content of Selected Foods (October 1986), and from Bowes and Church's "Food Values of Portions Commonly Used", 1985.
*Grams per 100 grams of food.

The above tables can only serve as a crude guide to lead you to natural foods which are high or low in complex carbohydrates and sugars. The estimates and blank spaces are due to the fact that the data aren't available. Dr. Frank Hepburn of the USDA informed me that the values for filling in blank spaces should be forthcoming within the next 20 years. However, even if they were available, your senses can tell you more now than these tables will tell you in 20 years.

For example, your senses tell you that as a fruit grows ripe, it becomes sweeter. This means that, for example, the high complex carbohydrate of a pear or a banana will break down to form more sugar as the fruit sets and ripens. Neither the data given above nor the data available in the future will be able to give you this information. Despite what the figures or estimates of fiber content are, only your body will be able to determine how much of the carbohydrate you eat will pass through without being absorbed (this is the definition of fiber) and how much you will use. And the amount of carbohydrate (and other food components) you digest will be different from what others may digest.

For these reasons, you must start listening to your body and realize that it can tell you things that "modern science" cannot. In time, as you proceed on the program, your body will be able to make the decisions on which foods you should eat at any given particular time without need for these tables.

Protein

Together with exercise, enzymes are important for the utilization of carbohydrates and fats as an energy source. Enzymes are proteins found in all living cells. They are responsible for catalyzing (or triggering) the chemical reactions that make life possible. These reactions lead to the breakdown of food to carbon dioxide, water, and urinary waste products; they produce the energy needed to support the life processes; they make possible the build-up of new tissues and the breakdown of old or unneeded tissues.

In the absence of enzymes, these reactions could not take place or could not take place at body temperature. For example, sugar is "burned" in the body at 98.6 degrees due to the action of enzymes, whereas sugar in a sugar bowl will not even begin to burn unless heated to over 250 degrees, a temperature far above the boiling point of water and a temperature at which life cannot exist.

Not until recently was it recognized that proteins and enzymes from food could be absorbed through the intestinal wall into the bloodstream. Antibody proteins from mother's milk are passed on through the intestinal wall of the infant intact, providing immunity to the child. In adults, enzymes, such as horseradish peroxidase, have been found to pass through the intestine intact. The fact that some of these enzymes pass through without any response by the immune system indicates that a tolerance to them may have been induced over the years and that these enzymes may play an important role (in some cases where this tolerance is not developed, food allergies occur and specific foods have to be removed from the diet). If enzymes do play an important role in the diet, then it is important that a substantial part your food should be eaten raw and as fresh as possible. You see, many enzymes are destroyed when the food they are in is cooked or processed.

Most proteins are broken down in the stomach and intestine to peptides or amino acids. Amino acids are the basic building blocks of proteins. When absorbed into the bloodstream, they are taken up by cells throughout the body which use them to make their own enzymes and structural proteins. The most predominant structural protein in the body is collagen, It makes up about 30% of your body's total amount of protein.

During exercise, the body increases the amount of breakdown of old structural proteins and enzymes and the build-up of new proteins and enzymes. The increases in lean body weight that result from the High Performance Health Program require an uptake of high quality protein. For nonvegetarians, I recommend a minimum of three units of animal protein daily. Units of animal protein are defined in the following table:

Units of Animal Protein

Units	Amount	Food	Protein Content
1	1 cup	milk	8-9 grams
1	1	egg	6-7 grams
1	1 ounce	cheese	6-7 grams
1	1 ounce	meat (trimmed)	5-6 grams
1	1 ounce	meat (from fish)	5-6 grams
1	1 ounce	liver, heart, or kidney	5-7 grams

In other words, someone eating:

(1) 3 eggs or
(2) one egg, one ounce of cheese, and one ounce of meat or
(3) 3 ounces of meat

would have three units of protein.

Starting off on the High Performance Health Program, I suggest those of you who have led a sedentary lifestyle to begin with 3-4 units of animal protein per day. Those who are more active, such as runners, swimmers, and cyclists should stay within 5-8 units, and those who are extremely active, such as serious weight-lifters, body builders, football players, professional athletes, should try to keep themselves to within 12 units of protein per day.

This does not mean that you must eat the exact same amount of animal protein each day. What it does mean is that over the course of a week, your average daily intake should fall within the suggested range.

If you start out on the program from a sedentary lifestyle, you will find that by keeping your animal protein consumption down to about four units per day, you will have little trouble reducing body fat and increasing lean body mass. As lean body mass increases and workouts become more strenuous, this protein intake will have to increase to meet the demands of (1) protein turnover to rejuvenate old muscles, tendons, ligaments, bones, etc., (2) protein accumulation to increase the mass of muscles, tendons, ligaments, and bones, and (3) protein synthesis within your body to provide it with the increased levels of enzymes, hemoglobin, hormones, and other proteins it needs.

However, eating excessive amounts of animal protein is an invitation to increasing body fat.

In general, intake of animal protein really appears to hold the key to the diet. The more you eat, the more your appetite seems to be fueled. For example, if you were to come over to my house for dinner and I served you two large baked potatoes, a large bowl of broccoli, and a large bowl of salad, you might find it very difficult to finish the meal. However, by adding 6 to 12 ounces of meat to the menu, I could probably get you to finish the whole meal. Since meat is so high in protein and contains virtually no carbohydrate, excessive meat consumption will lead you to take in excessive amounts of carbohydrate from other sources to balance off the high protein. This increased consumption of carbohydrates, unless burned off by increased activity levels, will be stored as fat.

Your diet will also contain additional protein from vegetable sources. This provides a useful addition of protein to the amount recommended above for animal protein. If you require increased levels of protein in your diet, it is wise to increase your intake of vegetable protein. The following table provides a list of the percentage of calories in various food groups that is present as protein.

Protein Content of Various Food Groups

Food	Protein Content
Meat (from lean fish)	70-95%
Organs (heart, liver, and kidney)	50-70%
Trimmed Meat	40-60%
Meat (from fatty fish)	40-50%
Eggs and Cheeses	20-40%
Whole "cow's" milk	30%
Untrimmed Meat	15-40%
Beans	20-30%
Nuts	15-20%
Grains and Seeds	10-20%

Values given as percent of the total caloric value of the food.

If you are a vegetarian, there is nothing stopping you from coming on the High Performance Health Program. If you are a strict vegetarian (no meat - no dairy - no eggs), you must get all your protein from vegetable products.

There are about 20 major amino acids which make up proteins and many other minor ones. Of the major amino acids, nine are considered essential. Some have claimed vegetable proteins are not rich enough in lysine and methionine, two of the nine essential amino acids. However, as you can see on the following table, there are a number of vegetarian foods that contain lysine or methionine levels higher than some animal products. Although these two tables contain the same information, their order is different. The first table contains foods listed in the order of decreasing lysine concentration. The second table contains foods listed in the order of decreasing methionine concentration. These tables show you some of the hazards of relying on soybean protein as a major vegetarian source of protein. (Text continues on page 85.)

Lysine and Methionine Contents of the Proteins of Various Foods
A. In the Order of Decreasing Lysine Content

FOOD	LYSINE	METHIONINE
Ricotta Cheese	10.3%	2.2%
Pork	9.9%	2.5%
Provolone Cheese	9.4%	2.4%
Mozzarella	9.2%	2.5%
Chicken Meat	9.0%	2.9%
Edam Cheese	9.0%	2.4%
Gouda Cheese	9.0%	2.4%
Turkey	8.9%	2.8%
Beef	8.7%	2.7%
Capon With Skin	8.6%	2.8%
Pork Tongue	8.6%	2.4%
Chicken With Skin	8.5%	2.8%
Capon	8.5%	2.8%
Cream Cheese	8.5%	2.3%
Neufchatel Cheese	8.5%	2.3%
Brick Cheese	8.5%	2.3%
Muenster Cheese	8.5%	2.3%
Romano Cheese	8.5%	2.5%
Parmesan Cheese	8.5%	2.5%
Roquefort Cheese	8.4%	2.5%
Feta Cheese	8.4%	2.5%
Sheep Milk Whole	8.4%	2.5%
Beef Tongue	8.3%	2.3%
Goat Milk Whole	8.3%	2.3%
Fontina Cheese	8.3%	2.5%
Swiss Cheese	8.3%	2.5%
Gruyere Cheese	8.3%	2.5%
Brie Cheese	8.3%	2.6%
Camembert Cheese	8.3%	2.7%
Beef Heart	8.3%	2.6%
Pork Heart	8.2%	2.5%

Lysine and Methionine Contents of the Proteins of Various Foods
A. In the Order of Decreasing Lysine Content
(continued)

FOOD	LYSINE	METHIONINE
Pork Spleen	8.1%	2.0%
Pork Brains	8.1%	2.1%
Blue Cheese	8.1%	2.5%
Pork Lungs	8.0%	1.8%
Adzuki Beans	**7.9%**	1.1%
Beef Spleen	7.9%	2.0%
Beef Lungs	7.8%	2.2%
Pork Pancreas	7.8%	1.9%
Pork Liver	7.7%	2.5%
Beef Tripe	7.7%	2.3%
Gjetost Cheese	7.7%	3.0%
Colby Cheese	7.7%	2.4%
Cheshire Cheese	7.7%	2.4%
Cheddar Cheese	7.7%	2.4%
Monterey Cheese	7.7%	2.4%
Caraway Cheese	7.7%	2.4%
Lentils	**7.6%**	0.9%
Chicken Giblets	7.6%	2.6%
Split Peas	**7.6%**	1.1%
"Cow" Milk	7.6%	2.4%
Port Du Salut Cheese	7.5%	2.8%
Limburger Cheese	7.5%	2.8%
Tilsit Cheese	7.5%	2.8%
Goose Egg Whole	7.3%	4.4%
Duck Egg Whole	7.3%	4.4%
Small White Beans	**7.3%**	1.6%
Pinto Beans	**7.3%**	1.6%
Cottage Cheese	7.3%	2.7%
Pork Kidneys	7.2%	2.2%
Black Beans	**7.2%**	1.6%
Black Turtle Beans	**7.2%**	1.6%

Lysine and Methionine Contents of the Proteins of Various Foods
A. *In the Order of Decreasing Lysine Content*
(continued)

FOOD	LYSINE	METHIONINE
Navy Beans	**7.2%**	1.6%
Yellow Bean	**7.2%**	1.6%
Kidney Beans	**7.2%**	1.6%
White Beans	**7.2%**	1.6%
Great Northern Beans	**7.2%**	1.6%
Pink Beans	**7.2%**	1.6%
Mung Beans	**7.2%**	1.2%
Beef Kidneys	7.1%	2.2%
Chickpeas	**6.9%**	1.4%
Beef Liver	6.9%	2.5%
Human Milk	6.9%	2.1%
Broadbeans	**6.9%**	0.9%
Black-eyes	**6.8%**	1.4%
Beef Brains	6.7%	2.3%
Baby Lima Beans	**6.7%**	1.3%
Lima Beans	**6.7%**	1.3%
Whole Hen Egg Frozen	6.6%	3.1%
Buckwheat*	**6.5%**	**2.4%**
Turkey Egg Whole	6.5%	3.1%
Quail Egg Whole	6.5%	3.1%
Pumpkin Seed	**6.5%**	**2.0%**
Pork Stomach	6.4%	2.1%
Soybeans	6.3%	1.3%
European Chestnut	5.9%	**2.3%**
Japanese Chestnut	5.6%	**2.1%**
Lotus Seeds	5.6%	1.5%
Pistachio Nuts	5.5%	1.6%
Chinese Chestnut	5.3%	**2.4%**
Poppy Seed	5.0%	**2.1%**
Fennel Seed	5.0%	**2.0%**
Chia Seeds	4.7%	**2.2%**

Lysine and Methionine Contents of the Proteins of Various Foods
A. In the Order of Decreasing Lysine Content
(continued)

FOOD	LYSINE	METHIONINE
Macadamia	4.2%	1.2%
Coconut	4.0%	1.7%
Rye*	3.8%	**2.2%**
Sunflower Seeds	3.7%	**2.0%**
Pine Nuts	3.6%	1.7%
Pecans	3.6%	**2.3%**
Peanuts	3.4%	0.9%
Hickorynuts	3.4%	**2.1%**
Brazilnuts	3.3%	**6.1%**
Safflower Seeds	3.1%	1.7%
Sesame Seeds	2.9%	**3.1%**
Black Walnuts	2.9%	**1.9%**
Almonds	2.9%	1.0%
Watermelon Seeds	2.8%	**2.6%**
English Walnuts	2.7%	**1.9%**
Wheat*	2.7%	**2.2%**
Filberts	2.6%	1.1%
Butternuts	2.5%	**2.0%**
Corn*	2.2%	**2.2%**
Barley*	2.0%	1.2%

Figures given as a percentage of the total major amino acids or approximately as a percentage of protein. The data on this table are derived from the U.S. Department of Agriculture's Computerized "Nutrient Data Base for Standard Reference, Release 5, Full Version".
*Estimates made based on data from Bowes and Church's "Food Values of Portions Commonly Used", 1985.
Boldface indicates proteins from vegetable sources that have a higher lysine or methionine content than one or more animal products.

Lysine and Methionine Contents of the Proteins
of Various Foods
B. In the Order of Decreasing Methionine Content

FOOD	METHIONINE	LYSINE
Brazilnuts	**6.1%**	3.3%
Goose Egg Whole	4.4%	7.3%
Duck Egg Whole	4.4%	7.3%
Turkey Egg Whole	3.1%	6.5%
Whole Hen Egg Frozen	3.1%	6.6%
Quail Egg Whole	3.1%	6.5%
Sesame Seeds	**3.1%**	2.9%
Gjetost Cheese	3.0%	7.7%
Chicken Meat	2.9%	9.0%
Capon With Skin	2.8%	8.6%
Capon	2.8%	8.5%
Chicken With Skin	2.8%	8.5%
Turkey	2.8%	8.9%
Tilsit Cheese	2.8%	7.5%
Limburger Cheese	2.8%	7.5%
Port Du Salut Cheese	2.8%	7.5%
Cottage Cheese	2.7%	7.3%
Beef	2.7%	8.7%
Camembert Cheese	2.7%	8.3%
Brie Cheese	2.6%	8.3%
Watermelon Seeds	2.6%	2.8%
Chicken Giblets	2.6%	7.6%
Beef Heart	2.6%	8.3%
Sheep Milk Whole	2.5%	8.4%
Roquefort Cheese	2.5%	8.4%
Feta Cheese	2.5%	8.4%
Pork Heart	2.5%	8.2%
Blue Cheese	2.5%	8.1%
Mozzarella	2.5%	9.2%
Fontina Cheese	2.5%	8.3%
Swiss Cheese	2.5%	8.3%

Lysine and Methionine Contents of the Proteins of Various Foods
B. In the Order of Decreasing Methionine Content
(continued)

FOOD	METHIONINE	LYSINE
Gruyere Cheese	2.5%	8.3%
Beef Liver	2.5%	6.9%
Pork	2.5%	9.9%
Pork Liver	2.5%	7.7%
Parmesan Cheese	2.5%	8.5%
Romano Cheese	2.5%	8.5%
Edam Cheese	2.4%	9.0%
Gouda Cheese	2.4%	9.0%
Provolone Cheese	2.4%	9.4%
Cheshire Cheese	2.4%	7.7%
Monterey Cheese	2.4%	7.7%
Cheddar Cheese	2.4%	7.7%
Colby Cheese	2.4%	7.7%
Caraway Cheese	2.4%	7.7%
"Cow" Milk	2.4%	7.6%
Chinese Chestnut	**2.4%**	5.3%
Pork Tongue	2.4%	8.6%
Buckwheat*	**2.4%**	**6.5%**
European Chestnut	**2.3%**	5.9%
Beef Tripe	2.3%	7.7%
Beef Brains	2.3%	6.7%
Goat Milk Whole	2.3%	8.3%
Pecans	**2.3%**	3.6%
Beef Tongue	2.3%	8.3%
Neufchatel Cheese	2.3%	8.5%
Cream Cheese	2.3%	8.5%
Brick Cheese	2.3%	8.5%
Muenster Cheese	2.3%	8.5%
Beef Kidneys	2.2%	7.1%
Beef Lungs	2.2%	7.8%
Ricotta Cheese	2.2%	10.3%

Lysine and Methionine Contents of the Proteins of Various Foods
B. In the Order of Decreasing Methionine Content
(continued)

FOOD	METHIONINE	LYSINE
Pork Kidneys	2.2%	7.2%
Chia Seeds	**2.2%**	4.7%
Wheat*	**2.2%**	2.7%
Corn*	**2.2%**	2.2%
Rye*	**2.2%**	3.8%
Poppy Seed	**2.1%**	5.0%
Human Milk	2.1%	6.9%
Pork Stomach	2.1%	6.4%
Japanese Chestnut	**2.1%**	5.6%
Pork Brains	2.1%	8.1%
Hickorynuts	**2.1%**	3.4%
Pork Spleen	2.0%	8.1%
Beef Spleen	2.0%	7.9%
Sunflower Seeds	**2.0%**	3.7%
Butternuts	**2.0%**	2.5%
Pumpkin Seed	**2.0%**	**6.5%**
English Walnuts	**1.9%**	2.7%
Black Walnuts	**1.9%**	2.9%
Pork Pancreas	1.9%	7.8%
Pork Lungs	1.8%	8.0%
Pine Nuts	1.7%	3.6%
Coconut	1.7%	4.0%
Safflower Seeds	1.7%	3.1%
Pistachio Nuts	1.6%	5.5%
Small White Beans	1.6%	**7.3%**
Pinto Beans	1.6%	**7.3%**
Kidney Beans	1.6%	**7.2%**
Black Turtle Beans	1.6%	**7.2%**
Great Northern Beans	1.6%	**7.2%**
Black Beans	1.6%	**7.2%**
Navy Beans	1.6%	**7.2%**

Lysine and Methionine Contents of the Proteins of Various Foods
B. In the Order of Decreasing Methionine Content
(continued)

FOOD	METHIONINE	LYSINE
Yellow Bean	1.6%	**7.2%**
Pink Beans	1.6%	**7.2%**
White Beans	1.6%	**7.2%**
Lotus Seeds	1.5%	5.6%
Black-eyes	1.4%	**6.8%**
Fenugreek Seed	1.4%	**7.0%**
Chickpeas	1.4%	**6.9%**
Soybeans	1.3%	6.3%
Baby Lima Beans	1.3%	**6.7%**
Lima Beans	1.3%	**6.7%**
Mung Beans	1.2%	**7.2%**
Macadamia	1.2%	4.2%
Barley*	1.2%	2.0%
Adzuki Beans	1.1%	**7.9%**
Filberts	1.1%	2.6%
Split Peas	1.1%	**7.6%**
Almonds	1.0%	2.9%
Lentils	0.9%	**7.6%**
Peanuts	0.9%	3.4%
Broadbeans	0.9%	**6.9%**

Figures given as a percentage of the total major amino acids or approximately as a percentage of protein. The data on this table are derived from the U.S. Department of Agriculture's Computerized "Nutrient Data Base for Standard Reference, Release 5, Full Version".

*Estimates made based on data from Bowes and Church's "Food Values of Portions Commonly Used", 1985.

Boldface indicates proteins from vegetable sources that have a higher lysine or methionine content than one or more animal products

Soybean protein is low in lysine and methionine and is usually sold as some highly processed trash product. My advice to strict vegetarians is — avoid soybean products and prepare your own foods from unprocessed ingredients. As you can see from the above table, most beans commonly cooked in the home have higher methionine and lysine contents. Simple recipes will be presented in the following chapter.

Although not normally considered a source of protein, 10-25% of the caloric value of vegetables is present as protein. The following table lists the lysine and methionine values of various vegetables, showing again that there is an ample amount of these amino acids in the vegetarian world. (Text continues on page 89.)

Lysine and Methionine Contents of the Proteins of Various Vegtables
A. In the Order of Decreasing Lysine Content

FOOD	LYSINE	METHIONINE
Mushrooms	10.4%	2.0%
Peas Edible Pod	8.5%	0.5%
Lambsquarters	8.5%	1.2%
Lettuce	7.6%	1.4%
Pea	7.4%	1.9%
Squash Summer	7.2%	1.9%
Squash Zucchini	7.2%	1.9%
Squash Crookneck	7.2%	1.9%
Watercress	7.2%	1.1%
Spinach	7.0%	2.1%
Pumpkin	7.0%	1.4%
Broccoli	6.9%	1.7%
Kale	6.7%	1.1%
Collards	6.6%	1.9%
Radishes	6.6%	1.3%
Cauliflower	6.5%	1.7%
Turnips	6.4%	2.0%
Turnip Greens	6.4%	2.2%
Onion	6.3%	1.1%
Garlic	6.2%	1.7%

Lysine and Methionine Contents of the Proteins of Various Vegtables
A. In the Order of Decreasing Lysine Content
(continued)

FOOD	LYSINE	METHIONINE
Leeks	6.2%	1.4%
Asparagus	6.1%	1.2%
Potatoes Flesh	6.1%	1.6%
Okra	6.0%	1.5%
Endive	5.8%	1.3%
Pepper	5.5%	1.5%
Seaweed Wakame	5.5%	**3.1%**
Seaweed Kelp	5.5%	1.7%
Pepper Hot Chili	5.5%	1.5%
Celery	5.4%	1.0%
Cucumber Raw	5.2%	0.9%
Seaweed Spirulina	5.2%	**2.0%**
Sweetpotato	5.1%	**2.6%**
Eggplant	5.0%	1.2%
Beet Greens	4.9%	1.4%
Taro	4.8%	1.4%
Yam	4.8%	1.7%
Beets	4.7%	1.5%
Cabbage	4.6%	1.0%
Squash Hubbard	4.5%	1.5%
Squash Butternut	4.5%	1.5%
Squash Spaghetti	4.5%	1.4%
Squash Winter	4.4%	1.5%
Squash Acorn	4.4%	1.5%
Tomato	4.3%	1.0%
Corn	4.2%	**2.0%**
Seaweed Laver	4.0%	**2.6%**

Figures given as a percentage of the total major amino acids or approximately as a percentage of protein. The data on this table are derived from the U.S. Department of Agriculture's Computerized "Nutrient Data Base for Standard Reference, Release 5, Full Version". Boldface indicates proteins from vegetable sources that have a higher lysine or methionine content than one or more animal products.

Lysine and Methionine Contents of the Proteins
of Various Vegtables
B. In the Order of Decreasing Methionine Content

FOOD	METHIONINE	LYSINE
Seaweed Wakame	3.1%	5.5%
Seaweed Laver	2.6%	4.0%
Sweetpotato	2.6%	5.1%
Turnip Greens	2.2%	6.4%
Spinach	2.1%	7.0%
Corn	2.0%	4.2%
Mushrooms	2.0%	10.4%
Seaweed Spirulina	2.0%	5.2%
Turnips	2.0%	6.4%
Pea	1.9%	7.4%
Squash Summer	1.9%	7.2%
Squash Zucchini	1.9%	7.2%
Squash Crookneck	1.9%	7.2%
Collards	1.9%	6.6%
Garlic	1.7%	6.2%
Yam	1.7%	4.8%
Cauliflower	1.7%	6.5%
Seaweed Kelp	1.7%	5.5%
Broccoli	1.7%	6.9%
Potatoes Flesh	1.6%	6.1%
Okra	1.5%	6.0%
Squash Acorn	1.5%	4.4%
Beets	1.5%	4.7%
Squash Hubbard	1.5%	4.5%
Squash Winter	1.5%	4.4%
Pepper Hot Chili	1.5%	5.5%
Pepper	1.5%	5.5%
Squash Butternut	1.5%	4.5%
Lettuce	1.4%	7.6%
Taro	1.4%	4.8%

Lysine and Methionine Contents of the Proteins of Various Vegtables
B. In the Order of Decreasing Methionine Content
(continued)

FOOD	METHIONINE	LYSINE
Leeks	1.4%	6.2%
Pumpkin	1.4%	**7.0%**
Squash Spaghetti	1.4%	4.5%
Beet Greens	1.4%	4.9%
Radishes	1.3%	**6.6%**
Endive	1.3%	5.8%
Asparagus	1.2%	6.1%
Eggplant	1.2%	5.0%
Lambsquarters	1.2%	**8.5%**
Onion	1.1%	6.3%
Kale	1.1%	**6.7%**
Watercress	1.1%	**7.2%**
Celery	1.0%	5.4%
Tomato	1.0%	4.3%
Cabbage	1.0%	4.6%
Cucumber Raw	0.9%	5.2%
Peas Edible Pod	0.5%	**8.5%**

Figures given as a percentage of the total major amino acids or approximately as a percentage of protein. The data on this table are derived from the U.S. Department of Agriculture's Computerized "Nutrient Data Base for Standard Reference, Release 5, Full Version". **Boldface** indicates proteins from vegetable sources that have a higher lysine or methionine content than one or more animal products.

Proteins provide three other functions.

(1) Glutamic acid and aspartic acid, two of the "nonessential amino acids" derived from the digestion of protein, can help support aerobic metabolism.

(2) Other amino acids are used to make nonprotein substances such as adrenalin, thyroxine, serotonin, and niacin.

(3) Proteins provide calories. During the building up of new body proteins and breaking down of old body proteins, a small percentage of the amino acid components are burned up to form carbon dioxide and water, and in the process, provide a small amount (about 10%) of the caloric energy used by your body. Eating excessive amounts of protein for use as an energy source increases the strain of having to detoxify the nitrogen that results from the use of protein for calories (in addition to having the drawback of stimulating an unnecessary increase in food intake as mentioned above).

Cofactors, coenzymes, catalysts, and performance enhancers

> *"In early times man . . . believed that strength and courage were endowed to those who ate the flesh of an especially brave animal. . . . ancient Greek, Roman, and Arab physicians . . . knew the therapeutic value of animal liver for the prevention or cure of night blindness. . . . In 1890 Eijkman, a Dutch physician, found that fowl fed almost exclusively on polished rice developed polyneuritic [nerve degeneration] symptoms . . . During 1890-1897 he was able to show that the disease disappeared when unmilled rice . . . [was] substituted for milled rice in the diet."*
>
> from *Vitamins and Coenzymes* by
> A. F. Wagner and K. Folkers

In order for enzymes to do their job, they often require dietary supplies of substances (cofactors, coenzymes, and catalysts) which your body cannot make. Some of these substances, such as riboflavin, pyridoxine, iron, magnesium, and zinc combine with enzymes to allow these enzymes to carry out their functions. Others, such as the essential amino acids and linoleic acid, provide some of the building blocks from which enzymes and other cell components are made. Still others, such as pantothenic acid or coenzyme A, tocopherols, and ascorbic acid, serve as catalysts which make possible some of the reactions necessary for life.

In addition, there are other substances which your body can make, but which can be more efficiently obtained through your diet. These include substances like niacin, hematin (organic iron), and omega-3 fatty acids. Since the dietary supply of these substances saves your body the unnecessary trouble of making them "from scratch", the efforts of your body can be directed to more worthwhile efforts. As a result, your performance improves. I call these substances "performance enhancers". As long as these substances are obtained from a balanced diet consisting of a wide variety of natural whole foods, you are safe. However, as soon as you start ingesting substances which have been fractionated from foods (such as testosterone or thyroxine) or eating inordinate amounts of exotic foods containing exceptionally high levels of these substances, you can expect trouble.

The substances discussed in this section include minerals (such as iron) and organic substances, such as ascorbic acid. Due to the short-sightedness of scientists in the past and their inability to admit they are wrong (this carries on to the present day), we have been stuck with the word "vitamin" to describe these organic substances. The term "vitamin" was originally coined to describe organic amine-containing (i.e. nitrogen-containing) substances necessary for life ("vita" is the Latin word for life). In fact, "vitamin" A contains no nitrogen, "vitamin" B3 is not necessary for life, "vitamin" C contains no nitrogen, and "vitamin" D contains no nitrogen and is not necessary for life.

The tragedy of this is that, for example, many people are taking "vitamin" D thinking it is essential to good health when it could be doing them harm (as it did to thousands of Englishmen when it was added to their milk supplies). In addition, the beneficial effects of many dietary substances have been neglected because, while they may be performance enhancers, they certainly cannot be classified as vitamins. Compounding the problem is that we have practitioners in the field giving nutritional advice and setting up diets who have been brought up with these misconceptions, who have no idea of the inadequacy of the information that they have been provided with, and who perpetuate these misconceptions to the general public.

You can get away from these problems by sticking with a diet composed of natural foods, processed or prepared as little and as gently as possible. If you want a diet rich in vital substances and performance enhancers, selection of foods from the following lists will safely provide you with these substances.

In addition, selection of these foods will help supply you with a balance. "Vitamins" often require the presence of minerals to be effective in carrying out their functions. For example, in some cases pyridoxine requires the presence of magnesium, ascorbic acid requires the presence of iron, and vitamin E requires the presence of selenium. More complicated associations exist between lipoic acid and glutathione, pantothenic acid (or coenzyme A), riboflavin, niacin, iron, cysteine, coenzyme Q, etc. Supplying one of these substances in pill form without the others limits its effectiveness. These requirements and associations are all preserved in unfractionated natural foods — and when you're eating these foods, you don't have to worry about whether or not you know the names of the chemicals they contain.

Many claim that "vitamins" and minerals in pill form are necessary because we cannot get enough from our diet. It is true that the typical Western diet does not provide enough "vitamins" and that minerals and supplements in pill form may solve some of the problems in people on these diets. However, a person living on a diet of coca cola and potato chips is not going to be helped much by taking vitamin pills. The only sound way to good health through nutrition is to start off with a nutritional foundation of good wholesome foods. (If you are going to use supplements, try to take the supplements along with foods that are rich in that particular supplement. In this way, you will be getting some of the factors necessary to help that supplement do its job.)

The U.S. National Academy of Sciences is the organization relied upon by the U.S. government for recommending how many calories as well as how much of each vitamin and mineral you should be ingesting daily. They refer to these values as Recommended Daily Allowances or RDAs. According to the National Academy of Sciences, you should be taking 1 RDA of each vitamin and mineral daily. The following table compares the average level of vitamins and minerals found in a reasonable 3000-calorie natural food diet (composed of 750 calories of fresh vegetables, 750 calories of fresh fruit, 500 calories of cereal grain, 250 calories of dry beans, 250 calories of dry nuts and seeds, and 500 calories of raw meat and eggs) with the amounts recommended by the National Academy of Sciences.

Nutritional Value of a Natural Food Diet.

Nutrient	RDAs in a Natural Food Diet	RDAs Recommended by the National Academy of Sciences
Vitamin A	7.7	1
Vitamin C	23.7	1
Vitamin B1	2.82	1
Vitamin B2	2.93	1
Vitamin B3	2.46	1
Vitamin B5	2.85	1
Vitamin B6	2.82	1
Vitamin Bc	4.92	1
Vitamin B12	2.04	1
Calcium	1.77	1
Iron	3.12	1
Magnesium	3.54	1
Phosphorus	2.61	1
Potassium	3.69	1
Sodium	0.69	1
Zinc	3.39	1
Copper	2.37	1
Manganese	3.93	1

A vegetarian diet comprised of 30% vegetable, 30% fruit, 12% grain, 20% beans, and 8% nuts & seeds would give similar results.

As you can see, the dietary vitamin and mineral intakes recommended by the National Academy of Sciences (with the exception of sodium) fall far short of the vitamin and mineral intakes provided by a reasonable diet. It almost looks like those responsible for setting the RDAs devised a good diet (similar to the one in the previous table) and divided the vitamin and mineral levels provided in the diet by three.

The levels of vitamins B1, B2, B3, B5, and B6 as well as iron, magnesium, phosphorus, potassium, zinc, copper, and manganese in the above diet are all about 3 times as high as the amount recommended by the National Academy of Sciences.

The level of vitamin A in this diet is about 8 times the amount recommended by the National Academy of Sciences. This is of special interest since numerous studies show that people eating diets high in vitamin A experience low cancer rates. Vitamin A is now being used in cancer therapy. The United States National Cancer Institute has become so interested in the beneficial effects of vitamin A that they have requested the United States Department of Agriculture to list in greater detail the vitamin A-like substances (called carotenoids) present in natural foods.

The level of vitamin C in this diet is about 20 times the amount recommended by the National Academy of Sciences. Many prominent scientists, including two-time Nobel-prize winner Linus Pauling, have long warned that the RDA for vitamin C was far too low. By substantially increasing dietary vitamin C intake, these investigators have reported success in preventing and reversing a number of degenerative diseases.

The level of calcium in the above diet is slightly higher than the amount recommended by the National Academy of Sciences and the level of sodium in this diet is on the low end of range recommended by the National Academy of Sciences.

In short, the amounts of vitamins and minerals recommended by the National Academy of Sciences, while adequate for preventing acute outbreaks of deficiency diseases in a majority of the people, are substandard and cannot be relied upon to reach and maintain a High Performance Health level.

Using the following tables in this chapter, you will be able to choose foods which will give you the greatest amount of vital substances and performance enhancers from your food in a minimum number of calories. The numbers used in these tables refer to the number of RDAs per 1000 calories. For example, in the following table, the value 45.00 means that 1000 calories of mustard spinach will supply you with 45 RDAs of vitamin A (i.e. 45 times the amount of vitamin A recommended by the U.S. National Academy of Sciences). The higher the number, the richer that food is in the particular nutrient listed. In most cases, the foods with the highest levels of vital substances are listed first with the remaining ones listed in declining order. While these foods are only evaluated on a limited number of known nutrients, the many other known and unknown vital substances and performance factors that are associated with them will also be provided by these foods.

Keep in mind that the purpose of the following tables is to show you which foods are highest in vital substances and performance enhancers, to support the statements that I make, and most important of all, to serve as a reference tool that you can use to help you select the foods you should eat. I would suggest that as you read this book for the first time, you read around the tables and refer to them only when the text refers you to them. In this way, you will find that you will be able to read this book more easily and more quickly. For this reason, I have indicated, before each long table, the page for you to go to so you can read around the tables and easily find the following text. (Text continues on page 105.)

Vitamin Contents of Raw Vegetables
(RDAs per 1000 Calories)

	Vitamin							
Vegetable	Vit. A	Vit. C	Vit. B1	Vit. B2	Vit. B3	Vit. B5	Vit. B6	Vit. Bc
Mustard Spinach	45.00	98.48	2.06	2.49	1.62	1.47	3.16	18.06
Vinespinach	42.11	89.47	1.75	4.80	1.39	0.51	5.7	18.43
Sweet Red Pepper	22.80	126.7	2.27	1.18	1.16	0.26	2.98	1.69
Pokeberry Shoots	37.83	98.55	2.32	8.44	2.75	0.39	2.89	1.72
Chrysanthium	86.35	36.27	1.22	7.72	2.66	0.47	3.48	11.25
Hot Chili Pepper	26.88	101.0	1.50	1.32	1.25	0.28	3.16	1.46
Watercress	42.73	65.15	5.46	6.42	0.96	5.12	5.33	2.09
Broccoli Leaves	57.14	55.48	1.55	2.50	1.20	3.47	2.58	6.34
Cabbage Pak- Choi	23.08	57.69	2.05	3.17	2.02	1.23	6.78	12.63
Swamp Cabbage	33.16	48.25	1.05	3.10	2.49	1.35	2.30	7.51
Sweet Pepper	2.12	85.33	2.27	1.18	1.16	0.26	2.90	1.69
Turnip Greens	28.15	37.04	1.73	2.18	1.17	2.56	4.43	18.00
Mustard Greens	20.39	44.87	2.05	2.49	1.62	1.47	3.15	18.02
New Zeal. Spinach	31.43	35.71	1.91	5.46	1.88	4.05	9.87	2.64
Chives	25.60	52.67	2.67	4.24	1.47	1.32	3.29	1.35
Spinach	30.55	21.29	2.36	5.05	1.73	0.54	4.03	22.09
Garden Cress	29.06	35.94	1.67	4.78	1.65	1.38	3.51	6.28
Broccoli Flowers	10.71	55.48	1.55	2.50	1.20	3.47	2.50	6.34
Parsley	15.76	45.45	1.62	1.96	1.12	1.65	2.26	13.87
Broccoli	5.50	55.48	1.55	2.50	1.20	3.47	2.58	6.34
Beet Greens	32.11	26.32	3.51	6.81	1.11	2.39	2.54	1.95
Carrots	65.42	3.61	1.50	0.81	1.14	0.83	1.55	0.81
Romain Lettuce	16.25	25.00	4.17	3.68	1.65	1.93	1.34	21.20
Broccoli Stalks	1.43	55.48	1.55	2.50	1.20	3.47	2.58	6.34
Lambsquarters	26.98	31.01	2.48	6.02	1.47	0.39	2.90	1.72
Scotch Kale	7.38	51.59	1.11	0.84	1.63	0.33	2.46	1.67
Cauliflower	0.08	49.65	2.11	1.40	1.39	1.07	4.38	6.89
Kale	17.80	40.00	1.47	1.53	1.05	0.33	2.46	1.47
Jute Potherb	16.35	18.14	2.61	9.45	1.95	0.39	8.02	9.04
Dock	18.18	36.36	1.21	2.67	1.20	0.34	2.52	1.50
Chicory Greens	17.39	17.39	1.74	2.56	1.14	9.16	2.08	11.90
Pumpkin Flowers	13.00	31.11	1.87	2.94	2.42	0.00	0.00	9.82
Pe-tsai Cabbage	7.50	28.13	1.67	1.84	1.32	1.19	6.59	12.30

Vitamin Contents of Raw Vegetables
(RDAs per 1000 Calories)
(continued)

				Vitamin				
Vegetable	Vit. A	Vit. C	Vit. B1	Vit. B2	Vit. B3	Vit. B5	Vit. B6	Vit. Bc
Seaweed Laver	14.86	18.57	1.87	7.50	2.21	2.71	2.07	10.45
Borage	20.00	27.78	1.91	4.20	2.26	0.36	1.82	1.57
Sesbania Flower	0.00	45.06	2.05	1.77	0.84	0.00	0.00	9.46
Spring Onion	20.00	30.00	1.87	3.29	0.42	1.05	1.11	1.37
Asparagus	4.09	25.00	3.46	3.32	2.72	1.44	3.16	13.57
Amaranth	11.23	27.76	0.69	3.58	1.33	0.45	3.36	8.20
Endive	12.06	6.37	3.14	2.60	1.24	9.63	0.54	20.88
Dandelion Greens	31.11	12.96	2.82	3.40	0.94	0.34	2.54	1.51
Chard Swiss	17.37	26.32	1.40	2.79	1.11	1.65	2.37	1.83
Tahitian Taro	5.13	40.00	1.03	3.59	1.31	0.56	1.32	0.57
Taro Leaves	11.50	20.63	3.32	6.39	1.90	0.36	1.58	7.48
Chicory Leaves	0.00	11.11	3.11	5.49	1.75	8.61	1.36	18.67
Beans Kidney Sprout	0.00	22.24	8.51	5.07	5.30	2.3	1.33	5.08
Cowpeas Leaf	2.45	20.69	8.14	3.55	2.03	0.38	2.77	8.73
Taro Shoots	0.45	31.82	2.42	2.67	3.83	1.24	4.59	0.75
Cabbage	0.54	35.42	1.39	0.74	0.66	1.06	1.80	5.91
Brussels Sprouts	2.05	32.95	2.16	1.23	0.91	1.31	2.32	3.54
Kohlrabi	0.15	38.27	1.24	0.44	0.78	1.11	2.53	1.49
Butterbur	0.36	37.50	0.95	0.84	0.75	0.42	3.12	1.86
Collards	17.53	20.44	1.02	1.98	1.04	0.61	1.60	1.51
Red Cabbage	0.15	35.19	1.24	0.65	0.59	2.18	3.54	1.92
White Icicle Radishes	0.00	34.52	1.43	0.84	1.13	2.39	2.44	2.55
Cabbage	0.54	32.85	1.39	0.74	0.66	1.06	1.80	5.91
Mushrooms	0.00	2.33	2.72	10.56	8.67	16.00	1.76	2.11
Celtuce	15.91	14.77	1.67	1.87	1.32	1.51	1.03	5.18
Looseleaf Lettuce	10.56	16.67	1.85	2.61	1.17	2.02	1.39	6.92
Lettuce Btrhd	7.46	10.26	3.08	2.72	1.22	2.52	1.75	14.10
Purslane	8.25	21.88	1.96	4.12	1.58	0.41	2.07	1.80
Pumpkin Leaves	10.21	9.65	3.30	3.96	2.55	0.40	4.95	4.76
Winged Bean Leaves	10.93	10.14	7.51	4.79	2.47	0.33	1.43	0.52
Savoy Cabbage	3.70	19.14	1.73	0.65	0.59	1.26	3.20	7.43
Coriander	13.85	8.75	2.47	3.53	1.92	1.68	2.39	1.29
Peas Edible Pod	0.33	23.81	2.38	1.12	0.75	3.25	1.73	2.48
Butternut Squash	17.33	7.78	1.48	0.26	1.40	1.62	1.56	1.48

Vitamin Contents of Raw Vegetables
(RDAs per 1000 Calories)
(continued)

				Vitamin				
Vegetable	**Vit. A**	**Vit. C**	**Vit. B1**	**Vit. B2**	**Vit. B3**	**Vit. B5**	**Vit. B6**	**Vit. Bc**
Radishes	0.06	22.35	0.20	1.56	0.93	0.94	1.90	3.97
Tomato	5.95	15.44	2.11	1.55	1.66	2.36	1.15	1.24
Scallop Squash	0.61	16.67	2.59	0.98	1.75	1.03	2.75	4.18
Black-eye Pea In Pods	3.64	12.50	2.27	1.87	1.44	3.91	1.79	2.98
Radish Sprouts	0.91	11.20	1.58	1.41	3.49	3.10	3.01	5.51
Waxgourd	0.00	16.67	2.05	4.98	1.62	1.86	1.22	1.00
Green Tomato	2.67	16.25	1.67	0.98	1.10	3.79	1.53	0.92
Oriental Radishes	0.00	20.37	0.74	0.65	0.59	1.39	1.16	3.92
Zucchini	2.43	10.71	3.33	1.26	1.50	1.08	2.89	3.95
Sweetpotato	19.11	3.60	0.42	0.82	0.34	1.02	1.11	0.33
Okra	1.74	9.25	3.51	0.93	1.39	1.17	2.57	5.78
Jew's Ear	0.00	0.40	2.16	4.80	0.15	14.47	1.60	1.91
Hubbard Squash	13.50	4.58	1.17	0.59	0.66	1.82	1.75	1.03
Iceberg Lettuce	2.54	5.00	2.36	1.36	0.76	0.64	1.40	10.77
Summer Squash	1.00	12.33	2.13	1.09	1.45	0.93	2.48	3.20
Winter Squash	10.97	5.54	1.75	0.43	1.14	1.97	1.01	1.47
Shallots	17.33	1.85	0.56	0.16	0.15	0.73	2.18	1.19
Welsh Onion	3.41	13.24	0.98	1.56	0.62	0.90	0.96	1.18
Bean Mung Sprout	0.07	7.33	1.87	2.43	1.31	2.30	1.33	5.07
Pumpkin	6.15	5.77	1.28	2.49	1.22	2.08	1.07	1.56
Lotus Root	0.00	13.10	1.91	2.31	0.38	1.22	2.09	0.57
Seaweed Wakame	0.80	1.11	0.89	3.01	1.87	2.82	0.02	10.86
Green Beans	2.16	8.76	1.81	1.99	1.28	0.55	1.09	2.94
Seaweed Spirulina	0.23	0.58	5.69	7.74	2.42	2.27	0.59	0.89
Dishcloth Gourd	2.05	10.00	1.67	1.77	1.05	1.98	0.98	0.84
Crookneck Squash	1.79	7.37	1.83	1.33	1.26	0.98	2.61	3.01
White-gourd Flower	0.14	12.02	1.38	0.92	1.20	1.97	1.30	1.05
Chayote Fruit	0.25	7.64	0.83	0.98	1.10	3.66	2.50	2.88
Turnips	0.00	12.96	0.99	0.65	0.78	1.35	1.52	1.34
Yellow Bean	0.35	8.76	1.81	1.99	1.28	0.55	1.09	2.94
Rutabagas	0.00	11.57	1.67	0.65	1.02	0.81	1.26	1.42
Cucumber	0.38	6.03	1.54	0.91	1.22	3.50	1.82	2.67
Alfalfa Sprouts	0.55	4.71	1.75	2.56	0.87	3.53	0.53	3.10
Seaweed Irish Moss	0.24	0.00	0.20	5.59	0.64	0.65	0.64	9.30

Vitamin Contents of Raw Vegetables
(RDAs per 1000 Calories)
(continued)

Vegetable	Vit. A	Vit. C	Vit. B1	Vit. B2	Vit. B3	Vit. B5	Vit. B6	Vit. Bc
Seaweed Kelp	0.28	0.00	0.78	2.05	0.58	2.72	0.02	10.47
Green Peas	0.79	8.23	2.18	0.96	1.36	0.23	0.95	2.01
Yardlong Bean	1.83	6.67	1.52	1.38	0.46	0.21	0.23	3.28
Broadbeans	0.49	7.64	1.57	0.90	1.10	0.22	0.24	3.34
Winged Beans	0.27	6.22	1.91	1.20	0.97	0.22	1.05	3.35
Celery	0.81	6.56	1.25	1.10	0.99	1.92	0.85	1.39
Bamboo Shoots	0.07	2.47	3.70	1.53	1.17	1.08	4.044	0.66
Squash Acorn	0.85	4.58	2.33	0.15	0.92	1.82	1.75	1.04
Yambean	0.00	8.13	0.65	0.43	0.39	0.22	0.24	3.35
Pigeonpeas	0.10	4.78	1.96	0.74	0.85	0.91	0.23	3.18
Beets	0.05	4.17	0.76	0.27	0.48	0.62	0.48	5.26
Artichokes	0.35	3.53	1.02	0.69	0.78	0.92	1.00	3.61
Hyacinth-beans	0.24	4.67	1.12	1.18	0.60	0.22	0.24	3.34
Seaweed Agar	0.00	0.00	0.13	0.50	0.11	2.11	0.56	8.15
Cassava	0.01	6.69	1.25	0.50	0.61	0.49	1.15	0.46
Celeriac	0.00	3.42	0.86	0.91	0.95	1.64	1.92	0.49
Cardoon	0.60	1.67	0.67	0.88	0.79	0.90	0.98	3.54
Onion	0.00	4.12	1.18	0.17	0.16	0.71	2.10	1.46
Pea Sprouts	0.13	1.35	1.17	0.71	1.27	1.46	0.94	2.81
Parsnips	0.00	3.78	0.80	0.39	0.49	1.46	0.55	2.23
Garlic	0.00	3.49	0.90	0.43	0.25	0.73	3.77	0.05
Leeks	0.16	3.28	0.66	0.29	0.35	0.42	1.74	2.63
Lentil Sprouts	0.05	2.59	1.43	0.71	0.56	0.99	0.82	2.36
Eggplant	0.27	1.03	2.31	0.45	1.22	0.57	1.64	1.69
Potato Flesh	0.00	4.16	0.74	0.26	0.99	0.88	1.50	0.41
Potato Skin	0.00	3.28	0.24	0.39	0.94	0.95	1.87	0.75
Lima Bean	0.27	3.45	1.28	0.54	0.69	0.40	0.82	0.75
Spaghetti Squash	0.15	1.06	0.75	0.32	1.52	1.98	1.39	0.91
Yellow Sweet Corn	0.33	1.32	1.55	0.41	1.04	1.61	0.29	1.33
White Sweet Corn	0.00	1.32	1.55	0.41	1.04	1.61	0.29	1.33
Salsify	0.00	1.63	0.65	1.58	0.32	0.82	1.54	0.80
Cowpeas	0.65	0.33	0.58	0.67	0.60	0.22	0.24	3.31
Jerusalem Artichokes	0.03	0.88	1.75	0.46	0.90	0.95	0.46	0.44
Chinese Waterchestnut	0.00	0.63	0.88	1.11	0.50	0.82	1.41	0.38

Vitamin Contents of Raw Vegetables
(RDAs per 1000 Calories)
(continued)

	Vitamin							
Vegetable	Vit. A	Vit. C	Vit. B1	Vit. B2	Vit. B3	Vit. B5	Vit. B6	Vit. Bc
Chinese Waterchestnut	0.00	0.63	0.88	1.11	0.50	0.82	1.41	0.38
Yam	0.00	2.42	0.63	0.16	0.25	0.48	1.13	0.49
Arrowhead	0.00	0.19	1.15	0.43	0.88	1.10	1.19	0.35
Chicory Roots	0.01	1.14	0.37	0.24	0.29	0.80	1.50	0.78
Eppaw	0.00	1.44	0.49	0.47	0.11	1.42	0.53	0.41
Burdock Root	0.00	0.69	0.09	0.25	0.22	0.81	1.52	0.79
Ginger Root	0.00	1.21	0.22	0.25	0.53	0.54	1.05	0.41
Rhubarb	2.33	0.00	0.48	6.35	0.63	0.84	0.75	0.74
AVERAGE	8.72	20.27	1.82	2.23	1.25	1.70	2.02	4.48

Mineral Contents of Raw Vegetables
(RDAs per 1000 Calories)

	Mineral								
Vegetable	Calcium	Iron	Magnesium	Phosphorus	Potassium	Sodium	Zinc	Copper	Manganese
Beet Greens	5.22	9.65	9.47	1.75	7.68	4.81	1.3	4.02	5.15
Spinach	3.75	6.84	8.98	1.86	6.76	1.63	1.6	2.36	10.19
Vinespinach	4.78	3.51	8.55	2.28	7.16	0.57	1.5	2.25	9.67
Purslane	3.39	6.91	10.63	2.29	8.23	1.28	0.7	2.83	4.73
Amaranth	6.89	4.96	5.29	1.60	6.27	0.35	2.3	2.49	8.51
New Zealand Spinach	3.45	3.18	6.96	1.67	2.48	4.22	1.8	2.66	11.41
Chard Swiss	2.24	5.26	10.66	2.02	5.32	5.10	1.3	3.77	4.82
Dock	1.67	6.06	11.70	2.39	4.73	0.08	0.6	2.38	3.97
Watercress	9.09	1.01	4.77	4.55	8.00	1.69	0.7	2.80	5.55
Borage	3.69	8.73	6.19	2.10	5.97	1.73	0.6	2.48	4.16
Chrysanthemum	2.75	10.23	2.50	1.57	8.96	1.39	0.8	3.27	5.46
Pumpkin Leaves	1.71	6.49	5.00	4.56	6.12	0.26	0.7	2.80	4.67
Seaweed Irishmoss	1.22	10.09	7.35	2.67	0.34	0.62	2.7	1.22	1.89
Jute Potherb	5.10	7.78	4.71	2.03	4.38	0.11	1.6	3.00	0.90

Mineral Contents of Raw Vegetables
(RDAs per 1000 Calories)
(continued)

Vegetable	Calcium	Iron	Magnesium	Phosphorus	Potassium	Sodium	Zinc	Copper	Manganese
Seaweed Wakame	2.78	2.69	5.94	1.48	0.30	8.81	0.6	2.52	7.78
Swamp Cabbage	3.38	4.88	9.34	1.71	4.38	2.70	0.6	0.48	2.11
Turnip Greens	5.86	2.26	2.87	1.30	2.92	0.67	0.5	5.19	4.32
Looseleaf Lettuce	3.15	4.32	1.53	1.16	3.91	0.23	1.1	0.98	10.42
Scotch Kale	4.07	3.97	5.24	1.23	2.86	0.76	0.6	2.31	3.86
Chicory Greens	3.62	2.17	3.26	1.70	4.87	0.89	1.2	5.13	4.66
Collards	5.13	1.81	2.24	0.70	2.08	0.67	3.4	5.47	4.86
Parsley	3.28	10.44	3.33	1.04	4.33	0.54	1.5	0.67	1.21
Mustard Spinach	7.96	3.79	1.25	1.06	5.44	0.43	0.5	1.36	4.63
Cabbage Pak-choi	6.73	3.42	3.65	2.37	5.17	2.27	1.0	0.65	3.06
Romain Lettuce	1.88	3.82	0.94	2.34	4.83	0.23	1.0	0.93	9.94
Seaweed Spirulina	0.39	5.96	1.83	0.35	1.30	1.71	0.5	9.19	1.79
Lambsquarters	5.99	1.55	1.98	1.40	2.80	0.46	0.7	2.73	4.55
Mustard Greens	3.30	3.12	3.08	1.38	3.63	0.44	0.5	2.26	4.62
Coriander	4.08	5.42	3.25	1.50	7.23	0.64	1.5	2.10	1.24
Endive	2.55	2.71	2.21	1.37	4.93	0.59	3.1	2.33	6.18
Butterbur	6.13	0.40	2.50	0.71	12.48	0.23	0.8	2.94	4.89
Seaweed Kelp	3.26	3.68	7.04	0.81	0.55	2.46	1.9	1.21	1.16
Seaweed Agar	1.73	3.97	6.44	0.16	2.32	0.16	1.5	0.94	3.59
Pokeberry Shoots	1.92	4.11	1.96	1.59	2.81	0.46	0.7	2.73	4.54
Mushrooms	0.17	2.76	1.00	3.47	3.95	0.07	2.0	7.87	1.12
Black-eye Pea Leaf	1.81	3.68	3.71	0.26	4.18	0.11	0.7	2.63	4.39
Seaweed Laver	1.67	2.86	0.14	1.38	2.71	0.62	2.0	3.02	7.06
Celtuce	1.48	1.39	3.18	1.48	4.00	0.23	0.8	0.73	7.82
Taro Leaves	2.12	2.98	2.68	1.19	4.11	0.03	0.7	2.57	4.25
Garden Cress	2.11	2.26	2.97	1.98	5.05	0.20	0.5	2.13	4.32
Okra	1.78	1.17	3.75	1.38	2.13	0.10	1.1	0.99	6.51
Chives	2.70	3.56	5.50	1.70	2.67	0.11	1.2	0.94	1.16
Taro Shoots	0.91	3.03	1.82	2.12	8.05	0.04	3.1	3.20	2.77
Chicory Witloof	1.00	1.85	2.17	1.17	3.24	0.21	2.8	2.08	5.52
Dandelion Greens	3.46	3.83	2.00	1.22	2.35	0.77	0.6	1.52	1.90
Cardoon	2.92	1.94	5.25	0.96	5.33	3.86	0.6	0.56	1.60
Jew's Ear	0.53	1.24	2.50	0.47	0.46	0.16	1.8	7.12	1.01
Rhubarb	7.10	3.41	0.58	1.43	0.56	3.66	0.9	0.03	0.40

Mineral Contents of Raw Vegetables
(RDAs per 1000 Calories)
(continued)

Vegetable	Calcium	Iron	Mag-nesium	Phos-phorus	Potas-sium	Sodium	Zinc	Copper	Man-ganese
Kale	2.25	1.89	1.70	0.93	2.38	0.39	0.6	2.32	3.87
Pe-tsai Cabbage	4.01	1.08	2.03	1.51	3.97	0.26	1.0	0.90	2.97
Zucchini	0.89	1.67	3.93	1.91	4.72	0.10	1.0	1.63	2.27
Asparagus	0.83	1.72	2.05	1.97	3.66	0.04	2.1	2.78	2.43
Spring Onion	2.00	4.20	2.00	1.10	2.74	0.07	1.2	0.96	1.17
White Icicle Radishes	1.61	3.18	1.61	1.67	5.33	0.52	0.6	2.83	0.59
Scallop Squash	0.88	1.24	3.19	1.67	2.70	0.03	1.1	2.27	2.18
Pumpkin Flowers	2.17	2.59	4.00	2.72	3.08	0.15	0.0	0.00	0.00
Alfalfa Sprouted	0.92	1.84	2.33	2.01	0.73	0.09	2.1	2.17	1.62
Crookneck Squash	0.92	1.40	2.76	1.40	2.98	0.05	1.0	2.15	2.07
Lettuce Btrhd	2.05	1.28	2.50	1.47	5.27	0.18	0.9	0.71	2.56
Potato Skin	0.43	3.10	0.99	0.55	1.90	0.08	0.4	2.92	2.60
Navy Bean Sprouts	0.19	1.60	3.77	1.24	1.22	0.09	0.9	2.13	1.52
Iceberg Lettuce	1.22	2.14	1.73	1.28	3.24	0.32	1.1	0.86	2.90
Broccoli Flower	1.43	1.75	2.23	1.96	3.10	0.44	1.0	0.64	2.05
Broccoli Leaves	1.43	1.75	2.23	1.96	3.10	0.44	1.0	0.64	2.05
Broccoli	1.43	1.75	2.23	1.96	3.10	0.44	1.0	0.64	2.05
Broccoli Stalks	1.43	1.75	2.23	1.96	3.10	0.44	1.0	0.64	2.05
Tahitian Taro	2.69	1.81	2.94	0.94	4.04	0.57	0.2	0.71	0.98
Summer Squash	0.83	1.28	2.88	1.46	2.60	0.05	0.9	1.52	1.96
Celery	1.88	1.67	1.88	1.35	4.73	2.50	0.7	0.88	2.13
Black-eye Peas In Pod	1.23	1.26	3.30	1.23	1.30	0.04	0.5	0.91	1.75
Radish Sprouts	0.99	1.11	2.56	2.19	0.53	0.06	0.9	1.12	1.51
Pinto Bean Sprouts	0.58	1.77	2.14	1.26	1.32	1.12	0.5	2.07	1.48
Mung Bean Sprouts	0.36	1.69	1.75	1.50	1.32	0.09	0.9	2.19	1.57
Bamboo Shoots	0.40	1.03	0.28	1.82	5.26	0.07	2.7	2.82	2.43
Oriental Radishes	1.25	1.24	2.22	1.07	3.36	0.53	0.6	2.56	0.53
Kidney Bean Sprouts	0.49	1.55	1.81	1.06	1.72	0.09	0.9	2.19	1.57
Green Beans	1.00	1.86	2.02	1.02	1.80	0.09	0.5	0.89	1.73
Yellow Beans	1.00	1.86	2.02	1.02	1.80	0.09	0.5	0.89	1.73
Cabbage Savoy	1.08	0.82	2.59	1.30	2.27	0.47	0.7	0.92	1.67
Red Cabbage	1.57	1.01	1.39	1.30	2.04	0.19	0.5	1.44	1.67
Artichokes	0.78	1.79	2.30	1.26	1.77	0.71	0.6	0.58	1.63
Peas Edible Pod	0.85	2.75	1.43	1.05	1.27	0.04	0.4	0.75	1.45

Mineral Contents of Raw Vegetables
(RDAs per 1000 Calories)
(continued)

Vegetable	Mineral								
	Calcium	Iron	Mag-nesium	Phos-phorus	Potas-sium	Sodium	Zinc	Copper	Man-ganese
Sweet Pepper	0.20	2.82	1.40	0.73	2.08	0.06	0.5	1.65	1.40
Sweet Red Pepper	0.20	2.82	1.40	0.73	2.08	0.06	0.5	1.65	1.40
Waxgourd	1.22	1.71	1.92	1.22	0.12	3.88	3.1	0.71	1.12
Pumpkin	0.67	1.71	1.15	1.41	3.49	0.02	0.8	1.95	1.20
Cauliflower	1.01	1.34	1.46	1.60	3.94	0.28	0.5	0.53	2.12
Chayote Fruit	0.66	0.93	1.46	0.90	1.67	0.08	1.0	2.05	1.97
Brussels Sprouts	0.81	1.81	1.34	1.34	2.41	0.26	0.7	0.65	1.96
Kohlrabi	0.74	0.82	1.76	1.42	3.46	0.34	0.1	1.91	1.29
Bean Lima	0.25	1.54	1.28	1.00	1.10	0.03	0.5	1.13	2.69
Hot Chili Pepper	0.38	1.67	1.56	0.96	2.27	0.08	0.5	1.74	1.48
Red Hot Chili Pepper	0.38	1.67	1.56	0.96	2.27	0.08	0.5	1.74	1.48
Cucumber	0.90	1.20	2.12	1.09	3.06	0.07	1.2	1.23	1.17
Eggplant	1.15	1.18	1.06	1.06	2.25	0.07	0.4	1.72	1.35
Celeriac	0.92	1.00	1.28	2.46	2.05	1.17	0.6	0.72	1.01
Red Tomato	0.31	1.40	1.45	1.01	2.91	0.19	0.4	1.62	1.61
Lotus Root	0.67	1.15	1.03	1.49	2.65	0.33	0.5	1.84	1.17
Cabbage	1.63	1.30	1.56	0.80	2.73	0.34	0.5	0.38	1.66
Cabbage	1.63	1.30	1.56	0.80	2.73	0.34	0.5	0.38	1.66
White-gourd Flower	1.55	0.79	1.96	0.77	2.86	0.07	3.3	0.74	1.18
Welsh Onion	0.44	1.99	1.69	1.20	1.66	0.23	1.0	0.82	1.01
Leeks	0.81	1.91	1.15	0.48	0.79	0.15	0.1	0.79	1.97
Winged Beans	1.43	1.70	1.74	0.63	1.21	0.04	0.5	0.42	1.11
Dishcloth Gourd	0.83	1.00	1.75	1.33	1.85	0.07	0.2	0.70	1.15
Lentil Sprouts	0.20	1.68	0.87	1.36	0.81	0.05	1.0	1.33	1.19
Garlic	1.01	0.63	0.42	0.86	0.72	0.05	0.5	0.80	2.81
Rutabagas	1.09	0.80	1.60	1.34	2.50	0.25	0.6	0.44	1.18
Hyacinth-beans	0.91	0.89	2.17	0.89	1.46	0.02	0.5	0.41	1.11
Yardlong Bean	0.89	0.56	2.34	1.05	1.36	0.04	0.5	0.41	1.09
Beets	0.30	1.15	1.19	0.91	1.96	0.74	0.6	0.76	2.00
Radishes	1.03	0.95	1.32	0.88	3.64	0.64	1.2	0.94	1.03
Green Tomato	0.45	1.18	1.04	0.97	2.27	0.25	0.2	1.50	1.04
Acorn Squash	0.69	0.97	2.00	0.75	2.31	0.03	0.2	0.65	1.04
Butternut Squash	0.89	0.86	1.89	0.61	2.09	0.04	0.2	0.64	1.12
Turnips	0.93	0.62	1.02	0.83	1.89	1.13	0.7	1.26	1.24

Mineral Contents of Raw Vegetables
(RDAs per 1000 Calories)
(continued)

Vegetables	Mineral								
	Calcium	Iron	Mag-nesium	Phos-phorus	Potas-sium	Sodium	Zinc	Copper	Man-ganese
Arrowhead	0.08	1.44	1.29	1.47	2.48	0.10	0.2	0.69	0.91
Broadbeans	0.26	1.47	1.32	1.10	0.93	0.32	0.5	0.41	1.11
Cassava	0.63	1.67	1.38	0.49	1.70	0.03	0.1	0.61	0.86
Green Pea	0.26	1.01	1.02	1.11	0.80	0.03	1.0	0.87	1.27
Winter Squash	0.70	0.87	1.42	0.72	2.52	0.05	0.2	0.70	1.14
Parsnips	0.40	0.44	0.97	0.79	1.33	0.06	0.5	0.64	1.87
Sprouted Peas	0.23	0.98	1.09	1.07	0.79	0.07	0.6	0.85	0.86
Jerusalem Artichokes	0.15	2.49	0.56	0.86	1.51	0.02	0.1	0.74	0.20
Eppaw	0.61	0.43	0.53	0.92	0.60	0.04	0.5	0.62	1.82
Ginger Root	0.22	0.40	1.56	0.33	1.60	0.09	0.3	1.31	0.83
Pigeonpeas	0.26	0.65	1.25	0.78	1.08	0.02	0.5	0.39	1.06
Sesbania Flower	0.59	1.73	1.11	0.93	1.82	0.25	0.0	0.00	0.00
Shallots	0.43	0.93	0.73	0.69	1.24	0.08	0.4	0.49	1.01
Burdock Root	0.48	0.62	1.32	0.59	1.14	0.03	0.3	0.43	0.81
Hubbard Squash	0.29	0.56	1.19	0.44	2.13	0.08	0.2	0.64	1.12
Carrots	0.52	0.65	0.87	0.85	2.00	0.37	0.3	0.44	0.83
Onion	0.61	0.61	0.74	0.71	1.22	0.03	0.4	0.47	0.98
Yambean	0.31	0.81	0.98	0.37	1.14	0.07	0.5	0.42	1.12
Potato Flesh	0.07	0.53	0.67	0.49	1.83	0.04	0.3	1.31	0.83
Salsify	0.61	0.47	0.70	0.76	1.24	0.11	0.3	0.43	0.82
Chicory Roots	0.47	0.61	0.75	0.70	1.06	0.31	0.3	0.42	0.80
Spaghetti Squash	0.58	0.52	0.91	0.30	0.87	0.23	0.4	0.45	0.95
Taro	0.34	0.29	0.77	0.65	1.47	0.05	0.1	0.64	0.90
Black-eye Peas	0.17	0.48	1.00	0.35	0.91	0.01	0.5	0.41	1.10
Chin. Waterchestnut	0.07	0.97	0.25	0.32	0.63	0.07	0.5	0.80	0.81
Chin. Waterchestnuts	0.09	0.03	0.52	0.50	1.47	0.06	0.3	1.23	0.78
Mountain Yam Hi	0.32	0.37	0.45	0.42	1.66	0.09	0.3	0.66	0.90
White Sweet Corn	0.02	0.34	1.08	0.86	0.84	0.08	0.4	0.25	0.47
Yellow Sweet Corn	0.02	0.34	1.08	0.86	0.84	0.08	0.4	0.25	0.47
Yam	0.12	0.25	0.45	0.39	1.84	0.04	0.1	0.60	0.84
Sweetpotato	0.18	0.31	0.24	0.22	0.52	0.06	0.2	0.64	0.85
AVERAGE	1.65	2.24	2.49	1.26	2.84	0.58	0.8	1.57	2.45

Although not particularly high on the list, items such as garlic, onions, and mushrooms appear to have particularly healthful properties due to substances that have not been fully characterized as yet and should be liberally incorporated into your diet.

As I have already pointed out, vegetables and fruits should be purchased fresh and eaten raw whenever possible. The vitamin contents of frozen vegetables and fruits are generally reduced. In particular, thiamin (vitamin B1) and ascorbic acid (vitamin C) are almost always reduced (by about 10-50%) in frozen fruits and vegetables.

In freezing vegetables, there is a loss of minerals from blanching and sometimes an uptake of sodium and other trace minerals from the water or the vessel they are processed in. Berries, the only fruits that are frozen on a large-scale basis, are not blanched and thus they retain most of their minerals during freezing. (Text continues on page 107.)

Vitamin Contents of Raw Fruits
(RDAs per 1000 Calories)

Fruit	Vitamin							
	Vit, A	Vit. C	Vit. B1	Vit. B2	Vit. B3	Vit. B5	Vit. B6	Vit. Bc
Acerola Cherries	2.41	873.7	0.42	1.10	0.66	1.76	0.13	
Guavas	1.55	59.97	0.65	0.58	1.24	0.53	1.27	
Currants, Euro. Black	0.37	47.88	0.53	0.47	0.25	1.15	0.48	
Papayas	15.49	26.41	0.46	0.48	0.46	1.02	0.22	
Strawberries	0.10	31.50	0.44	1.29	0.40	2.06	0.89	1.48
Orange W/peel	0.63	29.58	1.67	0.74	0.66	1.50	1.06	
Lemon	0.10	30.46	0.92	0.41	0.18	1.19	1.25	0.91
Cantaloup	9.20	20.10	0.69	0.35	0.86	0.66	1.49	1.21
Kiwifruit	0.30	26.78	0.22	0.48	0.43			
Grapefruit, Pink	0.87	21.17	0.76	0.39	0.34	1.72	0.64	1.02
Orange	0.45	18.87	1.23	0.50	0.32	0.97	0.58	1.61

Vitamin Contents of Raw Fruits
(RDAs per 1000 Calories)
(continued)

Fruit	Vitamin							
	Vit. A	Vit. C	Vit. B1	Vit. B2	Vit. B3	Vit. B5	Vit. B6	Vit. Bc
Rose-apples	1.36	14.87	0.53	0.71	1.68			
Grapefruit, White	0.03	16.82	0.75	0.36	0.43	1.56	0.59	0.76
Lime	0.03	16.17	0.67	0.39	0.35	1.32	0.65	0.68
Mullberries	0.07	14.11	0.45	1.38	0.76			
Tangerines	2.09	11.67	1.59	0.29	0.19	0.83	0.69	1.16
Jujube	0.05	14.56	0.17	0.30	0.60	0.47		
Mango	5.98	7.10	0.59	0.52	0.47	0.45	0.94	
Honeydew Melon	0.11	11.81	1.47	0.30	0.90	1.08	0.77	
Carambola	1.48	10.71	0.57	0.48	0.66			
Currants Red Or White	0.21	12.20	0.48	0.53	0.09	0.21	0.57	
Melon Casaba	0.12	10.26	1.54	0.45	0.81			
Kumquat	0.48	9.89	0.85	0.93	0.42			
Gooseberries	0.66	10.49	0.61	0.40	0.36	1.18	0.83	
Carissa	0.06	10.22	0.43	0.57	0.17			
Raspberries	0.27	8.50	0.41	1.08	0.97	0.89	0.53	1.33
Apricots	5.44	3.47	0.42	0.49	0.66	0.91	0.51	0.45
Guavas, Strawberry	0.13	8.94	0.29	0.26	0.46			
Watermelon	1.16	5.00	1.67	0.37	0.33	1.20	2.05	0.17
Sugar-apple	0.01	6.44	0.78	0.71	0.49	0.44	0.97	
Blackberries	0.31	6.73	0.38	0.45	0.40	0.84	0.51	1.63
Oheloberry	2.96	3.57	0.40	0.76	0.51			
Pricklypears	0.12	5.69	0.23	0.86	0.59			
Passion-fruit, Purple	0.72	5.15	0.00	0.79	0.81			
Pineapple	0.04	5.24	1.25	0.43	0.45	0.59	0.81	0.54
Cherry, Sour Red	2.56	3.33	0.40	0.47	0.42	0.52	0.40	0.38
Breadfruit	0.04	4.69	0.71	0.17	0.46	0.81		
Peach	1.26	2.56	0.26	0.56	1.21	0.72	0.19	0.20
Roselle	0.59	4.08	0.15	0.34	0.33			
Plums	0.58	2.88	0.52	1.03	0.48	0.60	0.67	0.10
Blueberries	0.18	3.87	0.57	0.53	0.34	0.30	0.29	0.29
Cranberry	0.10	4.59	0.41	0.24	0.11	0.81	0.60	0.09
Persimmon, Japanese	3.10	1.79	0.29	0.17	0.08		0.27	

Vitamin Contents of Raw Fruits
(RDAs per 1000 Calories)
(continued)

Fruit	Vitamin							
	Vit, A	Vit. C	Vit. B1	Vit. B2	Vit. B3	Vit. B5	Vit. B6	Vit. Bc
Nectarine	1.51	1.84	0.23	0.49	1.06	0.59	0.23	0.19
Loquat	3.26	0.35	0.27	0.30	0.20			
Grapes, European Type	0.10	2.54	0.86	0.47	0.22	0.06	0.70	0.14
Avocado, Florida	0.54	1.18	0.64	0.64	0.90	1.58	1.14	1.19
Sapotes	0.31	2.49	0.05	0.09	0.71			
Quinces	0.26	2.50	0.23	0.31	0.18	0.26	0.32	
Cherry, Sweet	0.29	1.62	0.46	0.49	0.29	0.32	0.23	0.15
Banana	0.09	1.65	0.33	0.64	0.31	0.51	2.86	0.52
Grapes, American Type	0.16	1.06	0.97	0.53	0.25	0.07	0.79	0.15
Jackfruit	0.32	1.19	0.21	0.69	0.22	0.52		
Avocado, California	0.34	0.74	0.41	0.41	0.57	1.00	0.72	0.93
Crabapple	0.05	1.75	0.26	0.15	0.07			
Tamarinds	0.01	0.24	1.19	0.37	0.43	0.11	0.13	
Apple	0.08	1.61	0.19	0.14	0.07	0.19	0.37	0.12
Pears	0.03	1.13	0.23	0.40	0.09	0.22	0.14	0.31
Figs	0.19	0.45	0.54	0.40	0.28	0.74	0.69	
AVERAGE	1.17	8.94*	0.6	0.52	0.52	0.8	0.73	0.6

*This excludes the value for acerola cherries

While a suitable alternative to candy and other sugar-laden junk foods, dry fruits suffer severe losses upon drying and should not be be substituted for fresh fruit. (Text continues on page 110.)

Vitamin Loss in Dried Fruits

Raw Fruit to Dry Fruit	Vitamin Loss				
	Vit. A	Vit. C	Vit. B1	Vit. B5	Vit. Bc
Apples To Dry Apples	73%	88%	54%	94%	
Apricots To Dry Apricots	36%	90%	87%	35%	84%
Currants To Dry Currants	67%	87%	19%	90%%	
Figs To Dry Figs	73%	88%	66%	58%%	
Peaches To Dry Peaches	47%	83%	84%	50%	74%
Pears To Dry Pears		61%	91%	51%%	
Plums To Dry Plums (prunes)		92%	56%	52%	74%
Grapes To Dry Grapes (raisins)	94%	88%	78%	29%	81%

Mineral Contents of Raw Fruits
(RDAs per 1000 Calories)

Fruit	Mineral								
	Calcium	Iron	Magnesium	Phosphorus	Potassium	Sodium	Zinc	Copper	Manganese
Roselle	3.66	1.68	2.60	0.63	1.13	0.06			
Pricklypears	1.14	0.41	5.18	0.49	1.43	0.06			
Mullberries	0.76	2.39	1.05	0.74	1.20	0.11	0.56		
Currant Red/white	0.73	1.36	0.95	0.78	1.36	0.01	0.3	0.5	1.02
Lemon	0.75	1.15	0.69	0.46	1.27	0.03	0.1	0.51	0.26
Melon Casaba	0.16	0.85	0.77	0.22	2.15	0.21			
Cantaloup	0.26	0.33	0.79	0.40	2.35	0.12	0.3	0.48	0.34
Currants Eur Black	0.49	0.99	0.58	0.65	1.31	0.01	0.3	0.76	0.83
Kiwifruit	0.36	0.37	1.23	0.55	1.45	0.04	0.0	0.00	0.00
Lime	0.92	1.11	0.50	0.50	0.91	0.03	0.2	0.87	0.07
Strawberries	0.39	0.70	0.83	0.53	1.48	0.02	0.3	0.65	2.42
Acerola Cherries	0.31	0.35	1.41	0.29	1.22	0.10			0.00
Blackberries	0.51	0.61	0.96	0.34	1.01		0.3	1.08	6.21
Passion-fruit Purple	0.10	0.92	0.75	0.58	0.96	0.13			
Loquat	0.28	0.33	0.69	0.48	1.51	0.01	0.1	0.34	0.79

Mineral Contents of Raw Fruits
(RDAs per 1000 Calories)

Fruit	Calcium	Iron	Magnesium	Phosphorus	Potassium	Sodium	Zinc	Copper	Manganese
Apricots	0.24	0.63	0.42	0.33	1.64	0.01	0.4	0.74	0.41
Rose-apples	0.97	0.16	0.50	0.27	1.31	0.00	0.2	0.26	0.29
Carissa	0.15	1.17	0.65	0.09	1.12	0.02		1.35	
Papayas	0.51	0.14	0.64	0.11	1.76	0.03	0.1	0.16	0.07
Gooseberries	0.47	0.39	0.57	0.51	1.20	0.01	0.2	0.64	0.82
Honeydew Melon	0.14	0.11	0.50	0.24	2.06	0.13		0.47	0.13
Guavas	0.33	0.34	0.49	0.41	1.48	0.03	0.3	0.81	0.71
Raspberries	0.37	0.65	0.92	0.20	0.83		0.6	0.60	5.17
Tamarinds	0.26	0.65	0.96	0.39	0.70	0.05			
Carambola	0.10	0.44	0.68	0.40	1.32	0.03	0.2	1.45	0.62
Jackfruit	0.30	0.35	0.98	0.32	0.86	0.01	0.3	0.80	0.52
Orange	0.71	0.12	0.53	0.25	1.03		0.1	0.38	0.13
Groundcherries	0.39	0.09	0.70	0.18	1.25		0.1	0.70	0.09
Grapefrt Pink/red	0.31	0.22	0.67	0.25	1.15		0.2	0.5	0.08
Watermelon	0.21	0.30	0.86	0.23	0.97	0.03	0.1	0.40	0.29
Avocado Florida	0.08	0.26	0.76	0.29	1.16	0.02	0.3	0.90	0.38
Breadfruit	0.14	0.29	0.61	0.24	1.27	0.01	0.1	0.33	0.15
Kumquat	0.58	0.34	0.52	0.25	0.83	0.04	0.1	0.68	0.34
Guavas Strawberry	0.25	0.18	0.62	0.33	1.13	0.24			
Quinces	0.16	0.68	0.35	0.25	0.92	0.03		0.91	
Banana Raw	0.05	0.19	0.79	0.18	1.15	0.00	0.1	0.45	0.41
Grapefrt White	0.27	0.12	0.61	0.27	1.03		0.1	0.35	0.14
Cherry Sour Red	0.27	0.36	0.45	0.25	0.92	0.03	0.1	0.83	0.56
Figs	0.39	0.28	0.57	0.16	0.84	0.01	0.1	0.38	0.43
Tangerines	0.27	0.13	0.68	0.19	0.95	0.01	0.4	0.25	0.18
Avocado California	0.05	0.37	0.58	0.20	0.96	0.03	0.2	0.6	0.34
Sugar-apple	0.21	0.35	0.56	0.28	0.70	0.04			
Peach	0.10	0.14	0.41	0.23	1.22		0.2	0.63	0.27
Nectarine	0.09	0.17	0.41	0.27	1.15		0.1	0.60	0.22
Sapotes	0.24	0.41	0.56	0.17	0.68	0.03			
Pineapple	0.12	0.42	0.71	0.12	0.61	0.01	0.1	0.90	8.41
Jujube	0.22	0.34	0.32	0.24	0.84	0.02	0.0	0.37	0.27

Mineral Contents of Raw Fruits
(RDAs per 1000 Calories)
(continued)

Fruit	Calcium	Iron	Magnesium	Phosphorus	Potassium	Sodium	Zinc	Copper	Manganese
Cherry Sweet	0.17	0.30	0.38	0.22	0.83		0.1	0.53	0.32
Oheloberry	0.21	0.18	0.54	0.30	0.36	0.02			
Grapes Amer Type	0.19	0.26	0.20	0.13	0.81	0.01	0.0	0.25	2.85
Crabapple	0.20	0.26	0.23	0.16	0.68	0.01	0.0	0.35	0.38
Plums	0.06	0.10	0.32	0.15	0.83		0.1	0.31	0.22
Grapes Euro Type	0.13	0.20	0.21	0.15	0.69	0.01	0.0	0.51	0.20
Mango	0.13	0.11	0.35	0.14	0.64	0.01		0.68	0.10
Pears	0.16	0.24	0.25	0.16	0.56		0.1	0.77	0.32
Persimmon Japanese	0.10	0.12	0.32	0.20	0.61	0.01	0.1	0.6	1.27
Cranberry	0.12	0.23	0.26	0.15	0.39	0.01	0.2	0.47	0.8
Apple	0.10	0.17	0.21	0.10	0.52			0.28	0.19
Blueberries	0.09	0.17	0.22	0.15	0.42	0.05	0.1	0.44	1.26
AVERAGE	0.36	0.45	0.71	0.30	1.07	0.04	0.2	0.58	0.88

Fruits are peculiar in containing high levels of citric acid and malic acid. Over 50% of the caloric value of lemons and limes is present in the form of citric acid. About 10% of the caloric values of currants and gooseberries is present in the form of citric acid. Citric acid and malic acid are used by the body in catalytic amounts to stimulate oxygen metabolism. While citric acid and malic acid can also be made by the breakdown of certain protein components, their inclusion in the diet in the form of fresh fruits should provide a performance-enhancing effect. (Text continues on page 112.)

Citric & Malic Acid Contents of Fresh Fruits

	Malic Acid	Citric Acid
Apple		0.5-1.0%
Apricots		1.0-2.0%
Banana		less than 0.5%
Blackberries	0.5-1.0%	
Blueberries	0.5-1.0%	
Cantaloup	less than 0.5%	
Carissa	1.0-2.0%	
Cherry Sour		1.0-2.0%
Cherry Sweet		0.5-1.0%
Crabapple		0.5-1.0%
Cranberry	2.0-3.0%	
Currants	2.0-3.0%	
Figs	less than 0.5%	
Gooseberries	2.0-3.0%	
Grapefruit	1.0-2.0%	
Groundcherries	1.0-2.0%	
Guavas	0.5-1.0%	
Jujube	less than 0.5%	
Kumquat	1.0-2.0%	
Lemon	over 3%	
Lime	over 3%	
Loquat	1.0-2.0%	
Mango	0.5-1.0%	
Mullberries		0.5-1.0%

Citric & Malic Acid Contents of Fresh Fruits
(continued)

Fruit	Citric Acid	Malic Acid
Nectarine		1.0-2.0%
Orange	1.0-2.0%	
Papayas	less than 0.5%	
Passion-fruit	2.0-3.0%	
Peach		0.5-1.0%
Pears	less than 0.5%	
Persimmon		less than 0.5%
Pineapple	0.5-1.0%	
Plums		1.0-2.0%
Pricklypears		less than 0.5%
Quinces		0.5-1.0%
Raspberries	1.0-2.0%	
Rose-apples	less than 0.5%	
Sapotes	less than 0.5%	
Strawberries	1.0-2.0%	
Sugar-apple	less than 0.5%	
Tangerines	1.0-2.0%	
Watermelon		less than 0.5%

* On a fresh weight basis

While not especially high in most vitamins, nuts and seeds do provide a good source of minerals, vitamin E, and high quality fats. All of the nuts and seeds in the following table can be and should be eaten raw. (Text continues on page 115.)

Vitamin Contents of Dry Nuts And Seeds
(RDAs per 1000 Calories)

Food	Vitamin								
	Vit. A	Vit. B1	Vit. B2	Vit. B3	Vit. B5	Vit. B6	Vit. Bc	Vit. C	Vit. E
Sunflower Seeds	0.01	2.68	0.26	0.42	2.15	0.61	1.00	0.04	7.86
Safflower Seeds	0.01	1.50	0.47	0.23	1.42	1.03	0.78	0.00	
Breadfruit Seeds	0.14	1.68	0.93	0.12	0.83	0.76	0.69	0.58	
Chestnut Japan	0.03	1.49	0.62	0.51	0.24	0.83	0.75	2.84	0.13
Lotus Seeds	0.02	1.29	0.27	0.25	0.47	0.86	0.78	0.00	
Peanuts	0.00	0.78	0.14	1.31	0.89	0.24	0.44	0.00	1.12
Chia Seeds	0.01	1.23	0.21	0.65	0.36	0.67	0.61	0.55	
Chestnut European	0.00	0.53	0.57	0.12	0.44	0.81	0.73	0.67	0.13
Chestnut Eur. Peeled	0.00	0.64	0.09	0.12	0.44	0.82	0.74	0.68	0.13
Pinyon	0.01	1.46	0.23	0.40	0.07	0.09	0.25	0.06	
Sesame Seeds	0.01	1.25	0.25	0.47	0.16	0.24	0.42	0.00	
Pistachio Nuts	0.04	0.95	0.18	0.10	0.37	0.20	0.25	0.21	0.89
Pine Nuts (pignolias)	0.01	1.05	0.22	0.36	0.07	0.10	0.28	0.06	
Hickorynuts	0.02	0.88	0.12	0.07	0.48	0.13	0.15	0.05	
Almonds	0.00	0.24	0.78	0.30	0.15	0.09	0.25	0.02	2.51
Pecans	0.02	0.85	0.11	0.07	0.47	0.13	0.15	0.05	0.22
Filberts	0.01	0.53	0.10	0.09	0.33	0.44	0.28	0.03	3.31
Filbert Blanch	0.01	0.51	0.10	0.09	0.32	0.43	0.28	0.02	3.31
Butternuts	0.02	0.42	0.14	0.09	0.19	0.42	0.27	0.09	
Almonds Blanch	0.00	0.18	0.68	0.28	0.14	0.08	0.16	0.02	2.51
Brazilnuts	0.00	1.02	0.11	0.13	0.07	0.17	0.02	0.02	0.99
Walnuts English	0.02	0.40	0.14	0.09	0.18	0.40	0.26	0.08	0.23
Pumpkin Seeds	0.07	0.26	0.35	0.17	0.11	0.19	0.27	0.06	
Walnut Black	0.05	0.24	0.11	0.06	0.19	0.41	0.27	0.09	
Watermelon Seeds	0.00	0.23	0.15	0.34	0.11	0.07	0.26	0.00	
Macadamia Nuts	0.00	0.33	0.09	0.16	0.11	0.13	0.06	0.00	
Coconut Dry	0.00	0.06	0.09	0.05	0.22	0.21	0.03	0.04	
Coconut Meat	0.00	0.12	0.03	0.08	0.15	0.07	0.19	0.16	0.20
AVERAGE	0.02	0.80	0.28	0.25	0.40	0.40	0.39	0.31	1.58

Mineral Contents of Dry Nuts and Seeds
(RDAs per 1000 Calories)

	Mineral								
	Calcium	Iron	Mag- nesium	Phos- phorus	Potas- sium	Sodium	Zinc	Copper	Man- ganese
Pumpkin Seeds	0.07	1.54	2.47	1.81	0.40	0.02	0.9	1.03	1.40
Breadfruit Seeds	0.16	1.07	0.71	0.76	1.31	0.06	0.3	2.40	0.19
Lotus Seeds	0.41	0.59	1.58	1.57	1.10	0.01	0.2	0.42	1.75
Chia Seeds	0.93	1.18	0.41	1.07	0.58	0.04	0.8	1.41	0.72
Sesame Seeds	0.60	0.74	1.22	1.05	0.20	0.02	0.9	1.49	0.73
Watermelon Seeds	0.08	0.73	2.31	1.13	0.31	0.08	1.2	0.49	0.72
Safflower Seeds	0.13	0.53	1.71	1.04	0.35	0.00	0.7	1.35	0.97
Sunflower Seeds	0.17	0.66	1.55	1.03	0.32	0.00	0.6	1.23	0.89
Pine Nuts (pignolias)	0.04	0.99	1.13	0.82	0.31	0.00	0.6	0.80	2.09
Chestnut Japan	0.17	0.52	0.80	0.39	0.57	0.04	0.5	1.46	2.58
Almonds Blanched	0.35	0.34	1.22	0.76	0.34	0.01	0.4	0.73	0.62
Almonds	0.38	0.35	1.26	0.74	0.33	0.01	0.3	0.64	0.96
Pistachio Nuts	0.19	0.65	0.68	0.73	0.51	0.00	0.2	0.82	0.14
Brazilnuts	0.22	0.29	0.86	0.76	0.24	0.00	0.5	1.08	0.29
Filberts	0.25	0.29	1.13	0.41	0.19	0.00	0.3	0.96	0.80
Filbert Blanched	0.24	0.28	1.10	0.40	0.18	0.00	0.2	0.93	0.78
Peanuts	0.09	0.32	0.79	0.56	0.34	0.01	0.4	0.71	0.49
Chestnut European	0.15	0.35	0.49	0.39	0.70	0.04	0.1	0.70	0.87
Chestnut Eur. Peeled	0.14	0.36	0.50	0.31	0.72	0.05	0.1	0.71	0.80
Walnut Black	0.08	0.28	0.83	0.64	0.23	0.00	0.4	0.67	1.76
Butternuts	0.07	0.36	0.97	0.61	0.18	0.00	0.3	0.29	2.68
Pinyon	0.01	0.30	1.03	0.05	0.29	0.06	0.5	0.73	1.91
Walnuts English	0.12	0.21	0.66	0.41	0.21	0.01	0.3	0.86	1.13
Hickorynuts	0.08	0.18	0.66	0.43	0.18	0.00	0.4	0.45	1.75
Pecans	0.04	0.18	0.48	0.36	0.16	0.00	0.5	0.71	1.69
Coconut Meat	0.03	0.38	0.23	0.27	0.27	0.03	0.2	0.49	1.06
Coconut Dry	0.03	0.28	0.34	0.26	0.22	0.03	0.2	0.48	1.04
Macadamia Nuts	0.08	0.19	0.41	0.16	0.14	0.00	0.2	0.17	0.21
AVERAGE	0.16	0.41	0.93	0.57	0.31	0.02	0.4	0.79	1.12

The following tables refer to the vitamin and mineral contents of meats derived from mammals (commonly referred to as "red meats"), fowl, shellfish, finfish, and others. The various meats in the "red" meat and fowl categories are listed in the order of decreasing vitamin B2 levels for vitamins and decreasing iron values for minerals.

Note how the B and C vitamin values as well as the mineral values are lower among untrimmed "red" meats and fowl meats with skin. This is because untrimmed meats or meat with skin on them have more fat. Since fat does not contain these water soluble nutrients, it adds more calories to the diet without increasing the levels of B vitamins, vitamin C, or minerals and thus lowers the amount of these nutrients on a per calorie basis. However, the fat content of these meats does increase their overall digestibility and you should include enough fat or skin with your meat to prevent the meat from tasting "dry". Moreover, fowl skin does increase the vitamin A values and most likely contains other fat soluble, performance enhancing nutrients.

Remember the old nursery rhyme:

> *Jack Sprat could eat no fat,*
> *His wife could eat no lean,*
> *But between the two of them,*
> *They licked the platter clean.*

Don't be like Jack Sprat or his wife. Try to steer a middle course and use your senses to determine the amount of fat or skin necessary to give the meat you eat a satisfying texture and taste. (Text continues on page 118.)

Vitamin Contents of Fresh "Red Meats"
(RDAs per 1000 Calories)

Food	Vitamin									
	Vit. A	Vit. C	Vit. B1	Vit. B2	Vit. B3	Vit. B5	Vit. B6	Vit. Bc	Vit. B12	Vit. E
Pork Trimmed	0.01	0.10	4.10	1.10	1.81	0.98	1.45	0.10	13.61	
Beef Trimmed			0.50	0.76	1.29	0.45	1.33	0.14	7.37	0.55
Pork Untrimmed	0.01	0.04	1.76	0.50	0.82	0.44	0.63	0.05	6.06	0.08
Lamb			0.37	0.43	0.91	0.36	0.50	0.05	2.70	0.40
Beef Untrimmed			0.21	0.32	0.55	0.19	0.57	0.05	3.22	0.80
AVERAGE	0.01	0.07	1.39	0.62	1.08	0.48	0.90	0.08	6.59	0.46

Mineral Contents of "Fresh Red Meats"
(RDAs per 1000 Calories)

Food	Mineral								
	Calcium	Iron	Magnesium	Phosphorus	Potassium	Sodium	Zinc	Copper	Manganese
Beef Trimmed	0.03	0.86	0.39	1.14	0.65	0.19	2.0	0.23	0.02
Pork Trimmed	0.04	0.39	0.39	1.27	0.65	0.20	1.1	0.22	0.02
Beef Untrimmed	0.02	0.36	0.16	0.48	0.26	0.09	0.8	0.10	0.01
Lamb	0.03	0.24	0.10	0.44	0.25	0.09	1.0	0.20	
Pork Untrimmed	0.02	0.17	0.17	0.57	0.29	0.09	0.5	0.10	0.01
AVERAGE	0.03	0.40	0.24	0.78	0.43	0.13	1.1	0.16	0.02

Vitamin Contents of Fowl
(RDAs per 1000 Calories)

Food	Vitamin								
	Vit. A	Vit. C	Vit. B1	Vit. B2	Vit. B3	Vit. B5	Vit. B6	Vit. Bc	Vit. B12
Quail Meat*	0.13	0.90	1.41	1.25	3.22	1.07	1.80	0.13	1.17
Squab Meat*	0.20	0.85	1.33	1.18	2.54	1.01	1.70	0.12	1.10
Quail Breast	0.09	0.69	1.30	1.16	3.51	1.16	1.96	0.08	1.27
Squab Breast	0.13	0.63	1.19	1.07	2.88	1.07	1.80	0.07	1.17
Turkey Leg	0.00	0.00	0.29	1.06	1.40	1.92	1.52	0.25	1.23
Pheasant Leg	0.43	0.75	0.35	0.92	1.45	1.30	2.51	0.19	2.09
Chicken Leg	0.18	0.41	0.41	0.87	2.63	1.82	1.20	0.20	0.96
Turkey Leg With Skin	0.01	0.00	0.24	0.86	1.16	1.54	1.20	0.19	1.03
Quail With Skin*	0.38	0.53	0.85	0.80	2.07	0.73	1.42	0.10	0.75
Duck Wild With Skin*	0.12	0.41	1.11	0.75	0.83	0.60	1.14	0.25	1.03
Turkey Breast	0.00	0.00	0.24	0.65	2.80	1.19	2.40	0.19	1.42
Pheasant Breast	0.33	0.75	0.41	0.53	3.39	1.31	2.53	0.08	2.11
Turkey Breast/skin	0.01	0.00	0.18	0.51	2.05	0.89	1.71	0.15	1.10
Chicken Breast	0.07	0.18	0.40	0.47	4.90	1.31	2.15	0.09	1.11
Pheasant With Skin*	0.29	0.49	0.27	0.46	1.87	0.93	1.66	0.08	1.42
Squab With Skin	0.25	0.29	0.48	0.45	1.08	0.47	0.63	0.05	0.45
Goose With Skin	0.05	0.19	0.15	0.39	0.51	0.63	0.48	0.03	0.31
Guinea Hen With Skin*	0.18	0.14	0.25	0.38	2.55	1.01	1.09	0.08	0.72
Chicken Leg With Skin	0.21	0.15	0.17	0.36	1.16	0.76	0.48	0.07	0.41
Capon With Skin*	0.16	0.12	0.18	0.32	1.64	0.75	0.70	0.06	0.48
Duck With Skin*	0.13	0.12	0.33	0.31	0.51	0.43	0.21	0.08	0.21
Chicken Breast/skin	0.16	0.08	0.21	0.27	2.52	0.78	1.17	0.05	0.61
AVERAGE	0.06	0.69	0.37	1.10	0.41	0.17	0.08	0.55	0.03

*includes both leg and breast;

Mineral Contents of Fowl
(RDAs per 1000 Calories)

	Mineral								
	Calcium	Iron	Mag-nesium	Phos-phorus	Potas-sium	Sodium	Zinc	Copper	Man-ganese
Quail Meat	0.08	1.87	0.47	1.91	0.47	0.17	1.3	1.77	0.04
Squab Meat	0.08	1.76	0.44	1.80	0.45	0.16	1.3	1.67	0.03
Quail With Skin	0.06	1.15	0.30	1.19	0.30	0.13	0.8	1.06	0.02
Duck Wild With Skin	0.02	1.10	0.24	0.66	0.31	0.12	0.2	0.59	0.02
Quail Breast	0.07	1.04	0.57	1.54	0.56	0.20	1.5	1.41	0.04
Squab Breast	0.06	0.96	0.52	1.42	0.52	0.19	1.3	1.29	0.03
Turkey Leg	0.10	0.83	0.50	1.28	0.59	0.28	1.6	0.58	0.05
Pheasant Leg	0.18	0.74	0.37	1.74	0.59	0.15	0.8	0.32	0.04
Turkey Leg With Skin	0.09	0.70	0.39	1.05	0.48	0.23	1.3	0.50	0.04
Squab With Skin	0.03	0.67	0.19	0.70	0.18	0.08	0.5	0.59	0.02
Turkey Breast	0.08	0.63	0.60	1.51	0.68	0.22	0.9	0.44	0.05
Turkey Breast/ Skin	0.08	0.51	0.45	1.14	0.51	0.17	0.7	0.36	0.04
Chicken Leg	0.08	0.46	0.46	1.08	0.47	0.31	1.1	0.20	0.04
Goose With Skin	0.03	0.37	0.12	0.53	0.22	0.09	0.3	0.29	0.01
Chicken Breast	0.09	0.36	0.59	1.37	0.56	0.27	0.6	0.14	0.04
Pheasant With Skin	0.06	0.35	0.28	0.99	0.36	0.10	0.4	0.14	0.02
Duck With Skin	0.02	0.33	0.09	0.29	0.14	0.07	0.2	0.23	0.01
Pheasant Breast	0.02	0.33	0.39	1.25	0.49	0.11	0.3	0.14	0.03
Guinea Hen With Skin	0.06	0.30	0.35	0.81	0.33	0.19	0.5	0.11	0.03
Capon With Skin	0.04	0.26	0.22	0.65	0.25	0.09	0.3	0.09	0.02
Chicken Breast/skin	0.05	0.24	0.31	0.73	0.29	0.16	0.3	0.09	0.02
Chicken Leg With Skin	0.04	0.23	0.20	0.48	0.20	0.14	0.4	0.09	0.02
AVERAGE	0.06	0.69	0.37	1.10	0.41	0.17	0.08	0.55	0.03

Notice how the vitamin B2 and iron levels of wild duck are 2 to 3 times higher than those of farm grown duck. Also notice how chicken, the most often consumed (and the most highly confined) fowl in the U.S., has the lowest vitamin B2 and iron values. And finally notice how the vitamin B2 and iron levels of fowl legs are greater than those of fowl breasts.

Increasing the activity of these animals stimulates the uptake and manufacture of substances which support these activities. If animals are allowed to walk and run around, the vitamin B2 and iron levels in their legs will increase, since these nutrients are essential for the aerobic metabolism which provides the energy necessary for continual output activities such as walking or running. Fowl breast, on the other hand is responsible for providing a quick burst energy to get the bird in the air. It gets this energy from anaerobic metabolism which requires magnesium and other factors, but does not require iron and vitamin B2. Therefore, the vitamin B2 and iron levels of fowl breast are lower than those of legs.

In practical terms, this shows us that we can expect to get greater nutritional value from the meat of animals that are allowed to roam and move around. It also means that if we want to gear our nutrition to support aerobic activities (long distance running, biking etc.), we should increase the proportion of fowl leg or dark meat that we eat. If however, we wish to improve our anaerobic capacity (for activities such as sprinting, heavy weight lifting etc.), we should increase the proportion of fowl breast or white meat in our diet. While I suggest a balance in white meat and dark meat as well as a balance in exercises requiring aerobic and anaerobic metabolism, there may be occasions in your life when you will be concentrating more on one than the other. It would be foolishness to do long aerobic workouts and not supply your body with the nutritional components to satisfy the demands of your body to increase its performance.

Remember, eating dark meat to stimulate aerobic metabolism does more than just give you vitamin B2 and iron, it gives you nutrients, which may not yet have been identified or whose importance may not yet have been recognized — and it gives you these nutrients in a balanced regimen.

Understanding this, we can begin to appreciate the primitive wisdom of our ancestors who "believed that strength and courage were endowed to those who ate the flesh of an especially brave animal."

The lack of detail on the shellfish, finfish, and "other" meat tables which follow is due to the current unavailability of data from the United States Department of Agriculture.

Vitamin Contents of Fresh "Shellfish"
(RDAs per 1000 Calories)

Food	Vit. A	Vit. C	Vit. B1	Vit. B2	Vit. B3	Vit. E
Oysters	1.22	6.53	1.14	1.38	1.37	0.93
Clammeat	0.41	2.28	0.91	1.37	0.94	
Mussel (meat)	0.32		1.12	1.30	0.72	
Snail Giant Afr.			0.09	0.97	1.01	
Squid			0.16	0.84	1.88	1.43
Abalone	0.31		1.22	0.84	0.70	
Snail			0.07	0.78	0.82	
Scallops	0.37		0.82	0.44	0.84	
Octopus			0.18	0.48	1.30	
Crayfish & Spinylobster			0.09	0.33	1.39	
Lobster Northern			2.93	0.32	0.87	1.62
Shrimp			0.15	0.19	1.85	
AVERAGE	0.51	4.41	0.81	0.86	1.13	1.27

Oysters, in addition to having the highest overall content of the vitamins listed on the above table, have very high values of vitamin B_{12}. Eating the liquid which accompanies the meat of clams and mussels increases the vitamin and mineral contents of these foods by about 50%. It is obvious that shellfish constitute a very important food source. Since they are very easily contaminated by water pollution, we have an additional reason to keep our waters unpolluted.

As can be seen from the following table, certain shellfish serve as a rich source of iron.

Mineral Contents of Fresh "Shellfish" (RDAs per 1000 Calories)

Food	Mineral				
	Calcium	Iron	Phosphorus	Potassium	Sodium
Oysters	0.98	4.51	1.60	0.42	0.43
Clammeat	0.79	4.41	1.97	0.83	0.75
Snail	0.11	2.66	3.11	1.40	0.44
Snail Giant Afr.	0.09	2.16	2.52	1.13	0.35
Mussel (meat)	0.77	1.99	2.07	0.88	1.38
Abalone	0.31	1.36	1.62	1.08	1.18
Scallops	0.27	1.23	2.14	1.30	1.43
Crayfish & Spinylobster	0.89	1.16	2.33	0.67	1.33
Shrimp	0.58	0.98	1.52	0.64	0.70
Octopus	0.33	0.53	1.97	1.33	0.46
Lobster Northern	0.27	0.37	1.68	0.53	1.05
Squid	0.12	0.33	1.18	1.15	0.40
AVERAGE	0.51	1.89	2.05	0.97	0.91

Finfish have exceptionally high levels of vitamin B3 which is probably the reason why they can put out a lot of energy for a reasonable length of time with limited supplies of oxygen. Because of the importance of finfish as a dietary source of vitamin B3, the following table lists various fish in the order of decreasing vitamin B3 concentrations. (Text continues on page 127.)

Vitamin Contents of Fresh "Finfish"
(RDAs per 1000 Calories)

			Vitamin			
Food	Vit. A	Vit. C	Vit. B1	Vit. B2	Vit. B3	Vit. E
Barracuda Pacific	0.24		0.24	0.52	6.19	
Tilefish	1.67		0.59	0.52	5.53	
Tuna Yellowfin	0.20		0.20	0.44	5.26	
Lingcod			0.40	0.28	5.20	0.36
Tautog	1.48		0.52	0.46	4.91	
Tuna Bluefin	0.19		0.18	0.41	4.83	
Sturgeon	1.40		0.50	0.44	4.65	
Rockfish	1.36		0.41	0.73	4.50	
Redhorse Silver	1.35			0.48	0.42	4.46
Halibut American	1.32		0.47	0.41	4.37	0.85
Bonito	0.16	0.50	0.16	0.35	4.17	
Albacore	0.15	0.47	0.15	0.33	3.95	
Swordfish	4.02		0.28	0.25	3.57	
Croaker	0.20		0.90	0.53	3.24	
Salmon Pink	0.58		0.78	0.25	3.18	
Dolly Varden (char)	0.23		0.28	0.25	3.07	
Halibut Greenland	0.90		0.05	0.28	2.99	
Dogfish Spiny	0.21		0.21	0.90	2.83	
Butterfish	0.20		0.59	0.84	2.62	
Shad	0.19		0.59	0.83	2.60	
Mackerel	0.47	0.29	0.32	1.12	2.58	0.88
Redfish		0.42	1.25	0.37	2.30	
Trout Rainbow	0.26		0.27	0.60	2.27	
Hake/whiting			0.90	1.59	2.13	
Salmon Sockeye	0.24		0.50	0.22	2.04	
Salmon Coho	0.37	0.09	0.32	0.35	2.04	
Salmon Chum	0.37		0.36	0.19	2.04	
Haddock			0.34	0.52	2.00	0.49
Red+gray Snapper			1.22	0.13	1.98	

Vitamin Contents of Fresh "Finfish"
(RDAs per 1000 Calories)
(continued)

Food	Vitamin					
	Vit. A	Vit. C	Vit. B1	Vit. B2	Vit. B3	Vit. E
Sablefish	0.49		0.39	0.28	1.94	2.29
Jack Mackerel	0.25		0.33	0.33	1.91	0.25
Chub	0.35		0.32	0.32	1.89	
Herring Pacific	0.31	0.51	0.14	0.96	1.88	1.09
Inconnu (sheefish)	0.35		0.32	0.32	1.87	
Grouper			1.30	0.47	1.81	
Lake Herring	0.31	0.52	0.63	0.61	1.81	
Salmon Atlantic	0.43	0.69	0.55	0.22	1.75	
Trout Brook	0.30	0.50	0.59	0.41	1.72	
Spot (croaker)	0.42		0.49	0.59	1.68	
Salmon Chinook	0.42		0.30	0.61	1.66	
Seabass White			0.69	1.23	1.64	
Cusk	0.24	0.44	0.27	0.63	1.61	
Tomcod Atlantic		0.43	0.52	1.30	1.50	
Cod		0.43	0.51	0.53	1.48	0.29
Spanish Mackerel	0.19	0.28	0.49	0.47	1.43	
Pike Northern	1.50		1.89	1.07	1.38	0.23
Pike Blue	1.47		1.85	1.05	1.35	0.22
Pike Walleye	1.42		1.79	1.01	1.30	0.22
Sardines Pacific	0.21	0.31	0.08	0.55	1.18	
Weakfish	0.25		0.50	0.29	1.17	
Pampano	0.20	0.30	1.65	0.78	1.14	
Flatfish (e.g. Flounder)			0.42	0.37	1.13	0.46
Bass White			0.68	0.18	1.13	
Ocean Perch			0.73	0.51	1.10	1.37
Herring Atlantic	0.19	0.28	0.08	0.50	1.08	0.61
Bass Black Sea			0.72	0.51	1.08	
Pickerel Chain	0.61	0.20	0.48	1.19	1.1	

Vitamin Contents of Fresh "Finfish"
(RDAs per 1000 Calories)
(continued)

Food	Vit. A	Vit. C	Vit. B1	Vit. B2	Vit. B3	Vit. E
Sauger (pike Var)	0.36	0.60	0.48	1.19	1.07	
Bullhead Black	0.36		0.32	0.21	1.07	
Bass Sm+lg/mouth			0.64	0.17	1.06	
Bass Striped			0.63	0.17	1.05	
Whitefish Lake	4.37		0.60	0.46	1.02	
Perch Yellow	0.33	0.55	0.44	1.10	0.98	
Burbot			3.17	1.00	0.96	
Crappie White	0.38	0.21		0.22	0.93	
Porgy+scup	0.27		0.71	0.47	0.89	
Pollock	1.39		0.35	0.62	0.89	0.33
Wreckfish	0.26		0.70	0.46	0.88	
Catfish	0.29		0.26	0.17	0.87	
Bluefish	0.26		0.68	0.45	0.85	
Kingfish	0.29	0.48	0.38	0.95	0.85	
Lake Trout	0.30		0.36	0.42	0.85	
Smelt Atlantic			0.07	0.72	0.75	
Yellowtail(pac.)	0.22		0.58	0.38	0.72	0.13
Buffalofish	0.45	0.15	0.06	0.21	0.70	
Sheepshead	0.45	0.15	0.06	0.21	0.70	
Carp	0.44	0.14	0.06	0.20	0.69	0.55
Smelt	0.43	0.14	0.23	0.20	0.67	
Perch White	0.43	0.14	0.06	0.20	0.67	
Alewife	0.40	0.13	0.05	0.19	0.62	
Suckers	1.27			0.40	0.61	
Sucker Carp	1.19			0.37	0.57	
Drum Freshwater	0.42	0.14	0.28	0.24	0.22	
AVERAGE	0.64	0.33	0.54	0.52	1.96	0.62

Mineral Contents of Fresh "Finfish"
(RDAs per 1000 Calories)

Food	Mineral				
	Calcium	Iron	Phos- phorus	Potas- sium	Sodium
Wreckfish	0.34	1.56	1.25	0.66	0.30
Jack Mackerel	0.05	0.82	1.60	0.78	0.24
Barracuda Pacific	0.12	0.79	1.40	0.69	0.16
Cusk	0.30	0.74	3.14	1.37	0.45
Herring Pacific	0.38	0.74	1.91	1.14	0.34
Chub	0.15	0.69	1.26	0.54	0.25
Inconnu (sheefish)	0.15	0.68	1.26	0.53	0.25
Sardines Pacific	0.17	0.63	1.12	0.70	0.21
Ocean Perch	0.18	0.61	1.89	0.95	0.35
Bass Black Sea	0.18	0.60	1.85	0.73	0.33
Bass White	0.17	0.57	1.80	0.70	0.32
Flatfish (e.g. Flounder)	0.13	0.56	2.06	1.15	0.45
Tuna Yellowfin	0.10	0.54	1.19	0.56	0.13
Bass Sm+lg/mouth	0.16	0.53	1.54	0.66	0.30
Bass Striped	0.16	0.53	1.68	0.65	0.29
Bonito	0.13	0.53	0.94	0.47	0.11
Hake/whiting	0.46	0.53	1.60	1.31	0.45
Mackerel	0.03	0.51	1.24	0.65	0.19
Albacore	0.12	0.50	0.89	0.44	0.10
Tuna Bluefin	0.09	0.50	1.09	0.51	0.12
Haddock	0.24	0.49	2.08	1.03	0.35
Tilefish	0.14	0.49	2.23	1.52	0.31
Red+gray Snapper	0.14	0.48	1.92	0.93	0.33
Burbot	0.23	0.47	1.93	0.99	0.34
Lingcod	0.13	0.46	2.09	1.37	0.32
Pickerel Chain	0.50	0.46	1.79	0.73	0.37
Grouper	0.22	0.45	1.89	0.93	0.32
Buffalofish	0.37	0.44	1.87	0.69	0.21
Sheepshead Atl.	0.37	0.44	1.45	0.55	0.41
Tautog	0.12	0.44	2.13	1.35	0.28
Carp	0.36	0.43	1.83	0.66	0.20
Perch White	0.35	0.42	1.36	0.65	0.19
Smelt	0.35	0.42	1.79	0.65	0.19

Mineral Contents of Fresh "Finfish"
(RDAs per 1000 Calories)
(continued)

Food	Mineral				
	Calcium	Iron	Phos- phorus	Potas- sium	Sodium
Swordfish	0.13	0.42	1.38	1.01	0.21
Crappie White	0.13	0.42	1.90	0.78	0.39
Sturgeon	0.12	0.41	1.87	1.27	0.26
Drum Freshwater	0.34	0.41	1.74	0.63	0.26
Pollock	0.11	0.41	1.85	0.98	0.23
Seabass White	0.36	0.41	1.23	1.01	0.35
Rockfish	0.11	0.40	1.81	1.07	0.28
Redhorse Silver	0.11	0.40	1.79	1.22	0.25
Sauger (pike Var)	0.12	0.40	1.79	0.73	0.37
Alewife	0.33	0.39	1.43	0.60	0.18
Halibut American	0.11	0.39	1.76	1.20	0.25
Suckers	0.10	0.37	1.76	0.86	0.24
Salmon Pink	0.89	0.37	1.67	0.69	0.24
Pampano	0.23	0.37	1.29	0.31	0.13
Perch Yellow	0.11	0.37	1.65	0.67	0.34
Salmon Sockeye	0.57	0.36	1.07	0.56	0.12
Sucker Carp	0.10	0.35	1.65	0.81	0.23
Herring Atlantic	0.21	0.35	1.21	0.64	0.19
Kingfish	0.10	0.32	1.43	0.63	0.36
Spanish Mackerel	0.33	0.31	1.17	0.40	0.17
Porgy+scup	0.40	0.30	1.86	0.68	0.26
Lake Herring	0.10	0.29	1.79	0.89	0.22
Tomcod Atlantic	0.11	0.29	2.10	1.32	0.41
Bluefish	0.16	0.28	1.73	0.96	0.29
Cod	0.11	0.28	2.07	1.31	0.41
Redfish	0.10	0.28	2.02	0.91	0.31
Weakfish	0.16	0.28	1.67	0.70	0.28
Trout Brook	0.10	0.28	2.19	0.84	0.21
Salmon Coho	0.78	0.27	1.03	0.60	0.12
Halibut Greenland	0.07	0.27	1.20	0.82	0.17
Bullhead Black	0.23	0.26	2.41	1.05	0.32
Lake Trout	0.13	0.26	1.18	0.46	0.22
Sablefish	0.35	0.26	1.32	0.50	0.13

Mineral Contents of Fresh "Finfish"
(RDAs per 1000 Calories)
(continued)

Food	Calcium	Iron	Phos-phorus	Potas-sium	Sodium
Pike Northern	0.12	0.25	2.03	0.97	0.26
Croaker	0.09	0.25	1.81	0.70	0.44
Pike Blue	0.12	0.25	1.98	0.95	0.26
Yellowtail(pac.)	0.14	0.24	1.47	0.81	0.24
Pike Walleye	0.12	0.24	1.92	0.91	0.25
Salmon Atlantic	0.30	0.23	0.71	0.52	0.16
Spot (croaker)	0.30	0.23	1.15	0.49	0.13
Trout Rainbow	0.11	0.23	1.02	0.40	0.19
Smelt Atlantic	0.09	0.23	2.31	1.04	0.32
Salmon Chinook	0.30	0.23	1.13	0.48	0.09
Catfish	0.19	0.22	1.97	0.85	0.26
Salmon Chum	0.57	0.21	1.07	0.62	0.13
Dolly Varden (char)	0.12	0.19	1.50	0.61	0.17
Dogfish Spiny	0.11	0.18	1.39	0.56	0.16
Butterfish	0.10	0.16	1.28	0.52	0.15
Shad	0.10	0.16	1.27	0.52	0.14
Whitefish Lake	0.14	0.14	1.45	0.51	0.15
AVERAGE	0.21	0.42	1.62	0.79	0.25

Of the organs listed in the following tables, tongue and heart are muscles. While not a skeletal muscle, tongue can legitimately be considered a meat. Its vitamin and mineral contents are virtually identical to meat. Heart, which is also a muscle, relies heavily on aerobic metabolism in order to carry out its functions. In order to support its increased aerobic needs, heart muscles have much higher levels of vitamin B2 and iron, as well as other substances that facilitate aerobic metabolism. By occasionally eating heart, even if you have to grind it along with beef for hamburger, you can provide an additional boost in the level of aerobic building blocks in your diet.

In addition to being high in all the B vitamins, liver (and, to a lesser extent kidney) provides an excellent source of iron, copper, vitamin A, vitamin C, and vitamin E, not to mention additional factors necessary for detoxification. I highly recommend the inclusion of liver in the diet at least once a week, preferably lamb liver or calf liver. To make it more appetizing, liver (or kidney) can also be ground into hamburger.

Vitamin Contents of Raw "Organs"
(RDAs per 1000 Calories)

	Vitamin									
Food	Vit. A	Vit. C	Vit. B1	Vit. B2	Vit. B3	Vit. B5	Vit. B6	Vit. Bc	Vit. B12	Vit. E
Beef Tongue		0.2	0.4	0.9	1.0	0.5	0.6	0.1	5.6	
Pork Tongue		0.3	1.5	1.3	1.2	0.5	0.5	0.0	4.2	
Pork Brains		1.8	0.8	1.3	1.8	4.0	0.7	0.1	5.7	
Beef Brains		2.2	0.8	1.3	1.9	1.8	0.9	0.1	28.8	
Pork Heart	0.1	0.7	3.5	5.9	3.0	3.9	1.5	0.1	10.7	
Beef Heart		0.9	1.1	5.1	4.3	3.6	1.7	0.0	38.9	0.5
Pork Liver	48.5	3.1	1.4	13.2	6.0	9.0	2.3	4.0	64.7	1.4
Beef Liver	74.2	2.6	1.2	11.4	4.7	9.7	3.0	4.3	161.3	0.5
Pork Kidneys	0.6	2.2	2.3	10.0	4.3	5.7	2.0	1.1	28.3	0.4
Beef Kidneys	2.5	1.4	2.4	14.0	3.9	6.2	2.2	1.9	84.2	0.2

Mineral Contents of Raw "Organs"
(RDAs per 1000 Calories)

	Mineral								
	Calcium	Iron	Mag- nesium	Phos- phorus	Potas- sium	Sodium	Zinc	Copper	Man- ganese
Beef Tongue	0.02	0.73	0.18	0.49	0.38	0.14	0.9	0.30	0.03
Pork Tongue	0.06	0.83	0.20	0.71	0.29	0.22	0.9	0.12	0.01
Pork Brains	0.07	0.70	0.28	1.85	0.54	0.43	0.7	0.76	0.19
Beef Brains	0.05	0.94	0.26	1.70	0.68	0.37	0.6	0.64	0.07
Pork Heart	0.04	2.20	0.40	1.19	0.66	0.22	1.6	1.38	0.13
Beef Heart	0.01	2.19	0.49	1.23	0.61	0.24	1.4	1.23	0.09
Pork Liver	0.06	9.66	0.34	1.79	0.54	0.30	2.9	2.02	0.64
Beef Liver	0.03	2.65	0.33	1.85	0.60	0.23	1.8	7.73	0.46
Pork Kidneys	0.08	2.72	0.43	1.70	0.61	0.55	1.8	2.49	0.31
Beef Kidneys	0.05	3.82	0.40	1.64	0.64	0.76	1.2	1.75	0.24

Eggs and beans, both good protein sources, also provide adequate amounts of vitamins and minerals. While both are short on vitamin C and while beans are short on vitamin A, these deficiencies are made up for by including fresh vegetables and fruit in the diet. (Text continues on page 132.)

Vitamin Contents of Raw Eggs
(RDAs per 1000 Calories)

	Vitamin								
Food	Vit. A.	Vit. B1	Vit. B2	Vit. B3	Vit. B5	Vit. B6	Vit. Bc	Vit. B12	Vit. E
Chicken Egg Whole	0.99	0.37	1.12	0.02	1.99	0.35	1.03	3.27	0.5
Chicken Egg Yolk	1.49	0.46	0.69	0.01	2.18	0.38	1.03	3.43	1.4
Chicken Egg White	0.00	0.07	3.44	0.10	0.90	0.03	0.81	0.44	0
Duck Egg Whole	2.15	0.56	1.28	0.06	1.83	0.61	1.08	9.70	
Goose Egg Whole	2.07	0.53	1.21	0.05	1.73	0.58	1.02	9.18	
Quail Egg Whole	0.57	0.55	2.93	0.05	2.02	0.43	1.05	3.32	
Turkey Egg Whole	0.97	0.43	1.62	0.01	2.01	0.35	1.04	3.30	
AVERAGE	1.18	0.42	1.76	0.04	1.81	0.39	1.01	4.66	0.63

Mineral Contents of Fresh Eggs
(RDAs per 1000 Calories)

Food	Mineral						
	Calcium	Iron	Magne-sium	Phos-phorus	Potas-sium	Sodium	Zinc
Chicken Egg Whole	0.30	0.74	0.19	0.95	0.22	0.40	0.6
Chicken Egg Yolk	0.34	0.84	0.10	1.15	0,07	0.06	0.6
Chicken Egg White	0.19	0.03	0.45	0.19	0.75	1.42	0.0
Duck Egg Whole	0.29	1.15	0.22	0.99	0.32	0.36	0.5
Goose Egg Whole	0.27	1.09	0.21	0.94	0.30	0.34	0.5
Quail Egg Whole	0.34	1.28	0.20	1.19	0.22	0.40	0.6
Turkey Egg Whole	0.48	1.33	0.20	0.83	0.22	0.40	0.6
AVERAGE	0.31	0.92	0.23	0.89	0.30	0.48	0.5

Vitamin Contents of Dry Beans
(RDAs per 1000 Calories)

Food	Vitamin							
	Vit. A.	Vit. C	Vit. B1	Vit. B2	Vit. B3	Vit. B5	Vit. B6	Vit. Bc
Black-eyes	0.01	0.07	1.69	0.40	0.33	0.81	0.48	4.71
Black Turtle	0.01	0.00	1.77	0.33	0.30	0.48	0.38	3.28
Black	0.01	0.00	1.76	0.33	0.30	0.48	0.38	3.26
Yellow	0.00	0.00	1.33	0.56	0.37	0.39	0.58	2.81
Split Peas	0.04	0.09	1.42	0.37	0.45	0.94	0.23	2.01
Pink	0.00	0.00	1.50	0.33	0.29	0.53	0.70	3.38
Broad	0.01	0.07	1.09	0.57	0.44	0.52	0.49	3.10
Small White	0.00	0.00	1.47	0.36	0.21	0.39	0.59	2.87
Navy	0.00	0.15	1.28	0.41	0.32	0.37	0.59	2.76
Gt Northern	0.00	0.26	1.28	0.41	0.30	0.59	0.60	3.55
Mung	0.03	0.23	1.19	0.39	0.34	1.00	0.50	4.50
Baby Lima	0.00	0.00	1.14	0.38	0.27	0.69	0.44	2.99

Vitamin Contents of Dry Beans
(RDAs per 1000 Calories)
(Continued)

Food	Vitamin							
	Vit. A.	Vit. C	Vit. B1	Vit. B2	Vit. B3	Vit. B5	Vit. B6	Vit. Bc
Kidney	0.00	0.23	1.06	0.39	0.33	0.43	0.54	2.96
Lentils	0.01	0.31	0.94	0.43	0.41	0.99	0.72	3.20
Adzuki	0.01	0.00	0.92	0.39	0.42			
Pinto	0.00	0.36	1.09	0.41	0.22	0.41	0.59	3.72
Lima	0.00	0.00	1.00	0.35	0.24	0.73	0.69	2.92
Chickpeas	0.02	0.18	0.87	0.34	0.22	0.79	0.67	3.82
White	0.00	0.00	0.87	0.26	0.08	0.40	0.43	2.91
AVERAGE	0.01	0.11	1.25	0.43	0.30	0.56	0.50	3.05

Mineral Contents of Dry Beans
(RDAs per 1000 Calories)

	Mineral								
	Calcium	Iron	Mag-nesium	Phos-phorus	Potas-sium	Sodium	Zinc	Copper	Man-ganese
White	0.60	1.74	1.43	0.75	1.44	0.02	0.7	1.18	1.35
Lima	0.20	1.23	1.66	0.95	1.36	0.02	0.6	0.88	1.24
Black Turtle	0.39	1.43	1.18	1.08	1.18	0.01	0.4	1.18	0.74
Small White	0.43	1.28	1.36	1.10	1.22	0.02	0.6	0.76	0.95
Black-eyes	0.27	1.37	1.37	1.05	0.88	0.02	0.7	1.01	1.14
Gt Northern	0.43	0.90	1.39	1.10	1.09	0.02	0.5	0.99	1.05
Kidney	0.36	1.37	1.05	1.02	1.13	0.03	0.6	1.15	0.77
Pink	0.32	1.10	1.33	1.01	1.14	0.01	0.5	0.94	1.00
Yellow	0.40	1.13	1.61	1.18	0.81	0.02	0.5	0.74	0.93
Navy	0.39	1.07	1.29	1.10	0.91	0.02	0.5	1.05	0.98
Broad	0.25	1.09	1.41	1.03	0.83	0.02	0.6	0.97	1.19
Baby Lima	0.20	1.03	1.40	0.92	1.12	0.02	0.5	0.79	1.26

Mineral Contents of Dry Beans
(RDAs per 1000 Calories)
(continued)

	Mineral								
	Calcium	Iron	Mag-nesium	Phos-phorus	Potas-sium	Sodium	Zinc	Copper	Man-ganese
Adzuki	0.17	0.84	0.97	0.97	1.02	0.01	1.0	1.33	1.31
Mung	0.32	1.08	1.36	0.88	0.96	0.02	0.5	1.08	0.75
Lentils	0.13	1.48	0.79	1.12	0.71	0.01	0.7	1.01	1.06
Pinto	0.30	0.96	1.17	1.02	1.04	0.01	0.5	0.91	0.83
Black	0.30	0.82	1.25	0.86	1.16	0.01	0.7	0.99	0.78
Chickpeas	0.24	0.95	0.79	0.84	0.64	0.03	0.6	0.93	1.51
Split Peas	0.13	0.72	0.84	0.89	0.77	0.02	0.6	1.02	1.02
AVERAGE	0.32	1.18	1.27	1.01	1.03	0.02	0.6	1.02	1.07

Whole grain cereals, which provide the bulk of the "staff of life" complex carbohydrates, also supply adequate amounts of most vitamins and minerals. While short on vitamin A, vitamin C, and calcium, these deficiencies can easily be made up for by inclusion of fresh vegetables and fruits in the diet. (Text continues on page 134.)

Vitamin Contents of Whole Grain Cereals
(RDAs per 1000 Calories)

	Vitamin							
Food	Vit. A.	Vit. B1	Vit. B2	Vit. B3	Vit. B5	Vit. B6	Vit. Bc	Vit. E
Wildrice	0.00	0.85	1.05	0.92				
Millet	0.00	1.49	0.68	0.37				
Wheat Durum	0.00	1.33	0.21	0.70				0.27
Buckwheat	0.00	1.19	0.26	0.69				
Wheat White*	0.00	1.05	0.21	0.83				0.30
Wheat Red	0.00	1.03	0.21	0.66				0.31
Oats	0.08	1.27	0.21	0.11	0.59	0.14	0.21	0.07

Vitamin Contents of Whole Grain Cereals
(RDAs per 1000 Calories)
(continued)

Food	Vit. A.	Vit. B1	Vit. B2	Vit. B3	Vit. B5	Vit. B6	Vit. Bc	Vit. E
Rye	0.00	0.86	0.39	0.25				
Rice Brown	0.00	0.63	0.08	0.69	0.54	0.64	0.11	0.42
Popcorn Unpopped	0.00	0.72	0.18	0.31				
Cornmeal White	0.00	0.71	0.18	0.30				0.04
Cornmeal Yellow	0.43	0.71	0.18	0.30				0.04
AVERAGE	0.042	0.987	0.322	0.51	0.565	0.393	0.161	0.206

Mineral Contents of Whole Grain Cerials

	Calcium	Iron	Magnesium	Phosphorus	Potassium	Sodium	Zinc	Copper	Manganese
Millet	0.05	1.16	1.24	0.79	0.35	0.00			
Wheat Durum	0.09	0.72		0.97	0.35	0.00			
Wildrice	0.04	0.66		0.80	0.17	0.01			
Rye	0.09	0.62		0.94	0.37	0.00			
Oats	0.11	0.61	0.96	1.03	0.24	0.00	0.05	0.36	2.36
Wheat Red	0.10	0.56		0.96	0.30	0.00			
Buckwheat	0.28	0.51		0.70	0.36	0.00			
Wheat White*	0.09	0.50		0.98	0.31	0.00			
Popcorn Unpopped	0.02	0.38		0.61	0.21	0.00			
Cornmeal White	0.05	0.38		0.60	0.21	0.00			
Cornmeal Yellow	0.05	0.38		0.60	0.21	0.00			
Rice Brown	0.07	0.25	0.61	0.51	0.16	0.01	0.73	0.23	1.13
AVERAGE	0.09	0.56	0.94	0.79	0.27	0.004	0.39	0.29	1.75

While it is advisable to stay away from sweeteners as much as possible, if you are going to use them, you might as well get some additional nutritional value out of them. The table below lists some of the sweeteners in the order of decreasing values of known nutrients. Note that besides calories, refined sugar, whether it is sucrose, glucose, or fructose, contains no nutritional value and should absolutely be avoided.

Vitamin & Mineral Contents of Various Sweeteners
(RDAs per 1000 Calories)

Food	Vitamin / Mineral							
	Vit.B1	Vit.B2	Vit.B3	Calcium	Iron	Phos- phorus	Potas- sium	Sodium
Malt Extract, Dried	0.65	0.72	1.41	0.11	1.32	0.67	0.17	0.10
Malt, Dry	0.89	0.50	1.29	0.11	0.60	0.67	0.17	0.10
Molasses, Blackstrap	0.34	0.52	0.49	2.68	4.20	0.33	3.66	0.20
Molasses, Medium	0.26	0.30	0.27	1.04	1.44	0.25	1.22	0.07
Molasses, Barbados	0.15	0.43	0.04	0.75	0.88	0.15	0.90	0.03
Sirup, Sorghum	0.34	0.23	0.02	0.56	2.70	0.08	0.18	0.02
Sirup, Maple	0.34	0.14	0.02	0.34	0.26	0.03	0.19	0.02
Sirup, Cane	0.33	0.13	0.02	0.19	0.76	0.09	0.43	0.01
Molasses, Cane Light	0.19	0.14	0.04	0.55	0.95	0.15	0.97	0.03
Honey	0.01	0.08	0.05	0.01	0.09	0.02	0.04	0.01
Sugars, Brown	0.02	0.05	0.03	0.19	0.51	0.04	0.25	0.04
Table Sugar (sucrose)	0.00	0.00	0.00	0.00	0.01	0.00	0.00	0.00
Dextrose	0.00	0.00	0.00	0.00	0.00	0.00	0.00	0.00
Fructose	0.00	0.00	0.00	0.00	0.00	0.00	0.00	0.00

The only dairy product you should drink is mothers milk, straight from the source — and if you're old enough to read this, chances are that its about time you started looking for other foods. From the tables below, you can see how different mothers milk is from the other milks listed. The high vitamin C level in mothers milk reflects the fact that while cows and other animals can make their own vitamin C, humans cannot, thus mothers milk must provide it for them. In addition, note the generally lower vitamin B levels and mineral levels of mothers milk. Mothers milk also differs in containing higher milk sugar levels and lower protein levels than other milks.

Those who feel they must consume dairy products to get enough calcium in their diet should refer back to the mineral composition table for vegetables. Vegetables provide abundant amounts of calcium. In the natural food diet presented near the beginning of this section, I included no dairy products, yet the diet contained more than adequate amounts of calcium.

Realizing however that nothing I say is going to stop you from occasionally "junking out" on dairy products, I urge you to at least stay away from all skim or low fat dairy products. While the tables below do not fully reflect it, these products are highest in the milk components that cause a majority of the milk related problems: lactose and milk proteins.

Vitamin Contents of Milk from Various Sources
(RDAs per 1000 Calories)

Food	Vitamin								
	Vit. A.	Vit. C	Vit. B1	Vit. B2	Vit. B3	Vit. B5	Vit. B6	Vit. Bc	Vit. B12
Human (mothers) Milk	0.92	1.20	0.13	0.30	0.13	0.58	0.07	0.19	0.22
Sheep Milk	0.39	0.64	0.40	1.94	0.20	0.69	0.25	0.16	2.20
Indian Buffalo Milk	0.55	0.39	0.36	0.82	0.05	0.36	0.11	0.15	1.25
Goat Milk Whole	0.81	0.31	0.47	1.18	0.21	0.82	0.30	0.02	0.32
3.7% Fat Whole Milk	0.53	0.38	0.40	1.48	0.07	0.89	0.20	0.12	1.85

Mineral Contents of Milk from Various Sources
(RDAs per 1000 Calories)

Food	Mineral						
	Calcium	Iron	Magne-sium	Phos-phorus	Potas-sium	Sodium	Zinc
Human (mothers) Milk	0.386	0.024	0.122	0.164	0.196	0.110	0.016
Sheep Milk	1.495	0.052	0.426	1.221	0.338	0.186	0.033
Indian Buffalo Milk	1.458	0.069	0.805	1.013	0.490	0.246	0.015
"Cows" Milk	1.545	0.043	0.522	1.209	0.627	0.346	0.039
Goat Milk	1.617	0.040	0.508	1.341	0.792	0.329	0.029

Vitamin Contents of Raw Milk and Cream Products
(RDAs per 1000 Calories)

Food	Vitamin								
	Vit. A.	Vit. C	Vit. B1	Vit. B2	Vit. B3	Vit. B5	Vit. B6	Vit. Bc	Vit. B12
Heavy Whipping Cream	1.22	0.03	0.04	0.19	0.01	0.13	0.03	0.03	0.17
Light Whipping Cream	1.01	0.03	0.05	0.25	0.01	0.16	0.04	0.03	0.22
Medium 25% Fat Cream	0.95	0.05	0.08	0.33	0.01	0.20	0.06	0.02	0.30
Sour Cream	0.91	0.07	0.11	0.41	0.02	0.31	0.03	0.13	0.47
Light Table Cream	0.93	0.06	0.11	0.45	0.02	0.26	0.07	0.03	0.38
Sour Half And Half	0.83	0.11	0.17	0.65	0.03	0.49	0.05	0.20	0.74
Half And Half Cream	0.82	0.11	0.18	0.67	0.03	0.40	0.14	0.05	0.84
3.7% Fat Whole Milk	0.53	0.38	0.39	1.48	0.07	0.89	0.30	0.19	1.85
3.3% Fat Whole Milk	0.50	0.25	0.41	1.55	0.07	0.93	0.31	0.20	1.94
Yogurt Plain (8g Protein/8oz)	0.49	0.14	0.31	1.36	0.06	1.15	0.24	0.30	2.02
Yogurt Lofat (11g Protein/8oz)	0.15	0.15	0.33	1.38	0.07	1.17	0.24	0.31	2.06
2% Lowfat Milk	1.15	0.32	0.52	1.95	0.09	1.17	0.39	0.26	2.44
Yogurt Lofat (12g Protein/8oz)	0.25	0.21	0.46	1.99	0.09	1.70	0.35	0.44	2.96
Buttermilk Cultured	0.20	0.40	0.56	2.24	0.08	1.24	0.38	0.31	1.81
1% Lowfat Milk	1.41	0.39	0.62	2.35	0.11	1.40	0.47	0.30	2.93
Skim Milk	1.75	0.47	0.69	2.36	0.13	1.71	0.52	0.37	3.61
Yogurt Skim (13g Protein/8oz)	0.04	0.26	0.57	2.47	0.12	2.09	0.43	0.55	3.66

Mineral Contents of Raw Milk and Cream Products
(RDAs per 1000 Calories)

Food	Calcium	Iron	Magnesium	Phosphorus	Potassium	Sodium	Zinc
Heavy Whipping Cream	0.156	0.005	0.051	0.151	0.058	0.050	0.004
Light Whipping Cream	0.198	0.006	0.062	0.174	0.088	0.053	0.006
Medium 25% Fat Cream	0.308	0.009	0.086	0.241	0.125	0.069	0.007
Light Table Cream	0.410	0.011	0.111	0.341	0.166	0.092	0.009
Sour Cream	0.453	0.016	0.131	0.330	0.179	0.113	0.008
Sour Half And Half	0.647	0.029	0.188	0.587	0.256	0.137	0.025
Half And Half Cream	0.670	0.030	0.195	0.608	0.265	0.142	0.026
3.7% Fat Whole Milk	1.545	0.043	0.522	1.209	0.627	0.346	0.039
Yogurt Plain (8g Protein/8oz)	1.638	0.045	0.471	1.288	0.671	0.343	0.064
3.3% Fat Whole Milk	1.619	0.045	0.547	1.267	0.658	0.363	0.041
Yogurt Lofat (11g Protein/8oz)	1.671	0.046	0.481	1.313	0.684	0.350	0.065
2% Lowfat Milk	2.040	0.056	0.688	1.596	0.829	0.457	0.052
Yogurt Lofat (12g Protein/8oz)	2.404	0.070	0.689	1.889	0.985	0.504	0.094
1% Lowfat Milk	2.449	0.066	0.825	1.915	0.994	0.548	0.062
Buttermilk Cultured	2.400	0.069	0.677	1.839	0.998	1.180	0.069
Yogurt Skim (13g Protein/8oz)	2.975	0.090	0.856	2.338	1.219	0.624	0.116
Skim Milk	2.946	0.064	0.814	2.409	1.265	0.671	0.076

In chapter 9, I present performance tests which you can apply to yourself to monitor your progress through the program. I guarantee that you will see a fall-off in your performance tests after consuming dairy products. Some of these problems may be avoided if you switch to cheese instead of milk. In the cheese-making process, the lactose which is present in milk is removed. The tables below provide the vitamin and mineral contents of most of the natural cheeses. (Text continues on page 140.)

Vitamin Contents of Natural Cheeses
(RDAs per 1000 Calories)

Food	Vit. A.	Vit. C	Vit. B1	Vit. B2	Vit. B3	Vit. B5	Vit. B6	Vit. Bc	Vit. B12
Feta Cheese	0.49	0.00	0.39	1.88	0.20	0.67	0.73	0.30	2.14
Gjetost Cheese	0.59	0.00	0.45	1.75	0.09	1.31	0.26	0.02	1.74
Lowfat 1% Cottage	0.15	0.00	0.19	1.34	0.09	0.54	0.43	0.43	2.91
Dry Curd Cottage	0.09	0.00	0.20	0.99	0.10	0.35	0.44	0.44	3.25
Lowfat 2% Cottage	0.22	0.00	0.18	1.21	0.08	0.49	0.39	0.37	2.65
Camembert Cheese	0.84	0.00	0.06	0.96	0.11	0.83	0.34	0.52	1.44
Creamed Cottage	0.46	0.00	0.14	0.93	0.06	0.37	0.29	0.30	2.01
Brie Cheese	0.55	0.00	0.14	0.92	0.06	0.38	0.32	0.49	1.65
Limburger Cheese	0.97	0.00	0.16	0.90	0.03	0.65	0.12	0.44	1.06
Whole Milk Tilsit	0.86	0.00	0.12	0.62	0.03	0.19	0.09	0.15	2.06
Blue Cheese	0.65	0.00	0.05	0.64	0.15	0.89	0.21	0.26	1.15
Roquefort Cheese	0.81	0.00	0.07	0.93	0.10	0.85	0.15	0.33	0.58
Port Du Salut Cheese	1.06	0.00	0.03	0.40	0.01	0.11	0.07	0.13	1.42
Edam Cheese	0.71	0.00	0.07	0.64	0.01	0.14	0.10	0.11	1.43
Provolone Cheese	0.75	0.00	0.04	0.54	0.02	0.25	0.09	0.07	1.39
Swiss Cheese	0.67	0.00	0.04	0.57	0.01	0.21	0.10	0.04	1.49
Part Skim Ricotta	0.82	0.00	0.10	0.79	0.03	0.32	0.07	0.24	0.70
Muenster Cheese	0.86	0.00	0.02	0.51	0.01	0.09	0.07	0.08	1.33
Gouda Cheese	0.49	0.00	0.06	0.55	0.01	0.17	0.10	0.15	1.44
Gruyere Cheese	0.73	0.00	0.10	0.40	0.01	0.25	0.09	0.06	1.29
Brick Cheese	0.81	0.00	0.03	0.56	0.02	0.14	0.08	0.14	1.13
Fontina Cheese	0.75	0.00	0.04	0.31	0.02	0.20	0.10	0.04	1.44
Skim Milk Mozzarella	0.70	0.00	0.05	0.70	0.02	0.06	0.13	0.09	1.07
Whole Milk Ricotta	0.77	0.00	0.05	0.66	0.03	0.22	0.11	0.18	0.65
Neufchatel Cheese	1.02	0.00	0.04	0.44	0.03	0.40	0.07	0.11	0.34
Cheddar Cheese	0.75	0.00	0.04	0.55	0.01	0.19	0.08	0.11	0.68
Monterey Cheese	0.68	0.00	0.03	0.61	0.01	0.10	0.10	0.12	0.74
Whole Milk Mozzarela	0.86	0.00	0.04	0.51	0.02	0.04	0.09	0.06	0.77
Parmesan Cheese	0.38	0.00	0.07	0.50	0.04	0.21	0.11	0.04	1.02
Cream Cheese	1.25	0.00	0.03	0.33	0.02	0.14	0.06	0.09	0.40
Romano Cheese	0.36	0.00	0.06	0.56	0.01	0.20	0.10	0.04	0.97
Colby Cheese	0.70	0.00	0.03	0.56	0.01	0.10	0.09	0.12	0.70
Cheshire Cheese	0.63	0.00	0.08	0.45	0.01	0.19	0.09	0.12	0.71
Caraway Cheese	0.77	0.00	0.05	0.70	0.03	0.09	0.09	0.12	0.24
AVERAGE	0.68	0.00	0.10	0.73	0.04	0.33	0.17	0.19	1.29

Mineral Contents of Natural Cheeses
(RDAs per 1000 Calories)

Food	Calcium	Iron	Magne-sium	Phos-phorus	Potas-sium	Sodium	Zinc
Parmesan Cheese	2.52	0.12	0.28	1.48	0.06	1.86	0.05
Romano Cheese	2.29	0.11	0.26	1.64	0.06	1.41	0.04
Swiss Cheese	2.13	0.03	0.24	1.34	0.08	0.31	0.07
Skim Milk Mozzarella	2.12	0.05	0.23	1.52	0.09	0.83	0.07
Gruyere Cheese	2.04	0.02	0.22	1.22	0.05	0.37	0.06
Provolone Cheese	1.79	0.08	0.20	1.18	0.10	1.13	0.06
Whole Milk Tilsit	1.72	0.04	0.10	1.23	0.05	1.01	0.07
Edam Cheese	1.71	0.07	0.21	1.25	0.14	1.23	0.07
Monterey Cheese	1.67	0.11	0.18	0.99	0.06	0.65	0.05
Part Skim Ricotta	1.64	0.18	0.27	1.10	0.24	0.41	0.06
Gouda Cheese	1.64	0.04	0.20	1.28	0.09	1.05	0.07
Muenster Cheese	1.62	0.06	0.19	1.06	0.10	0.77	0.05
Feta Cheese	1.56	0.14	0.18	1.07	0.06	1.92	0.07
Port Du Salut Cheese	1.54	0.07	0.17	0.85	0.10	0.69	0.05
Whole Milk Mozzarela	1.53	0.04	0.17	1.10	0.06	0.60	0.05
Brick Cheese	1.51	0.06	0.16	1.01	0.10	0.69	0.05
Roquefort Cheese	1.49	0.08	0.20	0.89	0.07	2.23	0.04
Cheddar Cheese	1.49	0.09	0.17	1.06	0.07	0.70	0.05
Caraway Cheese	1.49	0.09	0.15	1.09	0.07	0.83	0.05
Colby Cheese	1.45	0.11	0.16	0.97	0.09	0.70	0.05
Cheshire Cheese	1.38	0.03	0.13	1.00	0.07	0.82	0.05
Limburger Cheese	1.27	0.02	0.16	1.00	0.10	1.11	0.04
Blue Cheese	1.25	0.05	0.16	0.91	0.19	1.80	0.05
Fontina Cheese	1.18	0.03	0.09	0.74	0.04	0.93	0.06
Camembert Cheese	1.08	0.06	0.17	0.96	0.17	1.28	0.05
Whole Milk Ricotta	0.99	0.12	0.16	0.76	0.16	0.22	0.04
Gjetost Cheese	0.72	0.06	0.38	0.79	0.81	0.59	0.02
Lowfat 1% Cottage	0.70	0.11	0.18	1.54	0.31	2.55	0.03
Lowfat 2% Cottage	0.64	0.10	0.17	1.40	0.29	2.06	0.03
Creamed Cottage	0.48	0.08	0.13	1.06	0.22	1.78	0.02
Brie Cheese	0.46	0.08	0.15	0.47	0.12	0.86	0.05
Dry Curd Cottage	0.31	0.15	0.12	1.02	0.10	0.07	0.04
Neufchatel Cheese	0.24	0.06	0.07	0.44	0.12	0.70	0.01
Cream Cheese	0.19	0.19	0.05	0.25	0.09	0.38	0.01
AVERAGE	1.35	0.08	0.18	1.05	0.13	1.02	0.05

Activity

Your activities determine the type of diet necessary to provide a balance for you. However, for the proper functioning of your body, a balance of activities is also necessary. Your activities should include movements which involve as many parts of your body as possible. They should consist of power exercises, speed work, endurance exercises, stretching exercises, and nonlinear exercises.

(1) **power exercises**. These exercises are designed to increase strength by progressively increasing the weights used in weight-lifting workouts. As a result of these heavy weight workouts, muscle mass increases, cartilage thickness increases, tendons and ligaments become stronger, and the activity of osteoclasts (cells which break down old bone tissue) and osteoblasts (cells which build new bone tissue) increase, resulting in a stronger and rejuvenated skeletal system. Some of these gains can be attributed to the stimulation of testosterone secretion which occurs during heavy weight workouts. *These are the exercises that increase lean body weight.* As your lean body weight increases, the number of calories you burn at rest (your basal metabolism rate) increases, again allowing you to burn off more fat.

(2) **speed work**. *These exercises are designed to increase the body's ability to react or move quickly.* These exercises require you to move various parts of your body quickly for relatively short periods of time. Examples include running, jumping, throwing, and shadow-boxing. Because these exercises call for maximal coordinated output for short periods of time, improvement in speed work exercises will lead to an improved performance in power exercises and vice-versa.

(3) **endurance exercises**. *These are the exercises that burn fat off.* Sometimes referred to as "aerobic exercises", they are performed at a pace that can be carried on for a relatively long period of time. Ideally, to be effective in burning off body fat, these exercises should last for at least 45 minutes to one hour. Workouts for 60 minutes are at least three times as effective in burning off body fat as 30 minute workouts. These exercises

include running, cycling, swimming, stair-climbing, and intensive lighter weight workouts. As a result of these exercises, hemoglobin, myoglobin, and cytochrome levels increase, allowing the body to increase its oxygen capacity. It is very important to combine endurance exercises with power exercises to build up the muscles, cartilage, ligaments, tendons, and bones so that they are able to withstand the longer-term stress and wear that they will receive during these extended workouts. In addition, speed workouts are necessary to allow you run, bike, etc. faster once your oxygen consumption capacity is no longer the limiting factor during your endurance workouts.

(4) **stretching exercises**. *These exercises are designed to* stretch muscles out in order to increase and *maintain flexibility and range of motion.* Some power, speed work, and endurance exercises cause muscles to contract and can result in a reduced amount of flexibility. On the other hand, a person engaged in excessive stretching without power, speed work, and/or endurance exercises can, in the extreme, look like a marionette with its strings cut.

(5) **nonlinear exercises**. Most of the above exercises rely on body movements along a straight line (linear) and do not provide much side to side (nonlinear) motion. Tennis, volleyball, and basketball are a few of the activities which develop coordination and build up those body parts that are used in nonlinear activities.

The following table lists some physical activities and an approximate evaluation of each with regard to the type of exercise they provide.

Activity	Power	Speed	Endurance	Stretching	Nonlinear
Running					
sprints	E	E	F	F	P
middle distances	G	G	G	F	P
long distances	F	F	E	P	P
Bicycling					
sprints	E	E	F	P	P

Activity	Power	Speed	Endurance	Stretching	Nonlinear
Bicycling					
medium distances					
in high gear	E	G	G	P	P
in low gear	G	E	E	P	P
long distances	F	F	E	P	P
Swimming					
sprints	E	E	G	G	F
medium distances	G	G	E	G	F
long distances	F	F	E	F	F
Weight-lifting					
(1 hour workout)					
high weight-low rep	E+	E	P	P	P
mid weight-mid rep	E	G	G	F	P
low weight-high rep	G	G	E	F	P
Stretching and yoga	P	P	P	E+	F
Rowing	E	E	E	F	P
Jumping and jump roping	E	E	F	F	P
Tennis	G	G	G	F	E
Shadow-boxing	G	E	G	P	F
Wrestling	E	E	G	E	E
Volleyball	G	G	G	G	G
Basketball	G	E	E	G	E
Dancing	F	F	G	F	F

E=excellent, G=good, F=fair, P=poor

To get you started, I have designed a basic exercise program which works out a number of different muscle groups and provides elements of power, endurance, and flexibility in a minimum amount of time. To begin the program, you must set aside 60 to 90 minutes three days a week (e.g. Sunday, Tuesday, and Thursday or Monday, Wednesday, and Friday). The session can be done in the early morning, late afternoon, or evening to fit around your schedule. Try not to eat in the two to three hours preceding your workout. If it is an absolute necessity that you eat during this period of time, eat some fruit like an apple, orange, or a piece of melon. Make sure you start out with an adequate of water in your body at the beginning of your workout and keep water (preferably distilled and definitely not fluoridated) on hand during the workout.

As you begin the program, the first thing to concentrate on is developing your form. By developing proper form, you will get the full advantage of each activity in the program and minimize your chances of getting injured. Second, try to cut down on the time it takes to go through the workout, but don't do this at the expense of your form. Take enough time to allow yourself the full benefit of each motion, but try to cut back on the time you rest between each workout activity. Finally, in activities involving weights, try to gradually increase the poundage of the weights you use.

While exercising, *don't forget to breathe.* When exerting force, some have a tendency to hold their breath. Although I will be suggesting, on some exercises, when to breathe in (when you are exerting maximum force) and when to breathe out (during the opposite motion), the most important thing you can do is just make sure you keep on breathing at a comfortable rate, even if you don't follow my specific instructions. In particular, at times you may wish to pick up your breathing rate to a level in excess of what I have suggested. By all means, let yourself breathe at an accelerated rate in these cases.

The Basic Exercise Program that follows is suitable for everyone from a beginner to a trained athlete. It is designed to provide the best combination of strength, endurance, and stretching exercises using as many muscle groups as possible in a relatively short period of time. I highly recommend that this basic program be supplemented with any of the activities which are listed in the table as having good to excellent "speed work" and/or "nonlinear exercise" ratings.

The Basic Exercise Program

Five Minute Warmup: Get on an exercise bicycle, make sure the seat is adjusted properly (when your pedal is pressed as far down as it can go, you should still have a slight bend in your

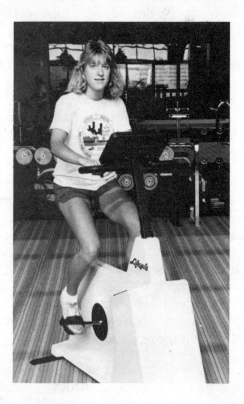

knee) and start pedaling. Try to keep up a speed of 60-90 revolutions of the crank per minute for 10 minutes. If you reach a speed of 90 revolutions per minute (rpm) and feel it is too easy, you can adjust the bike to make it harder to pedal. The idea of this warmup is to get your aerobic metabolism up to a reasonably high rate. By proceeding quickly throughout the workout, you can maintain this high rate of aerobic metabolism as a base. For this reason, I suggest that between each exercise, no more than 45 seconds be taken to stretch and recover.

Exercise #1. Toe Raises — place your toes and the balls of your feet on a three inch high platform (or a stair step) and slowly raise your heels until you are standing on your tiptoes. Then

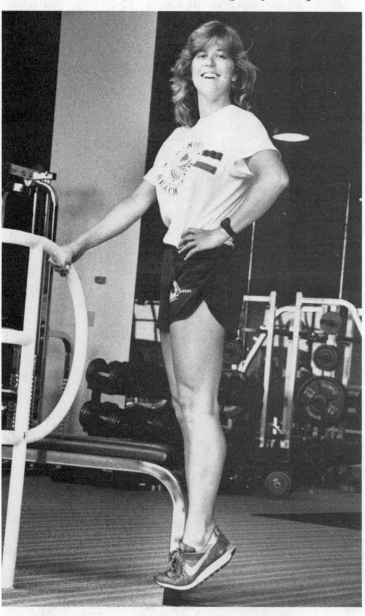

slowly allow your heels to come down as low as possible. From this position, raise your heels to a tiptoe position. Perform this motion 10 times or as many times as you can up to 10 times and stop. If this is too easy, do your toe raises 10 times with one foot and 10 times with the other foot. Take up to 30 seconds for recovery.

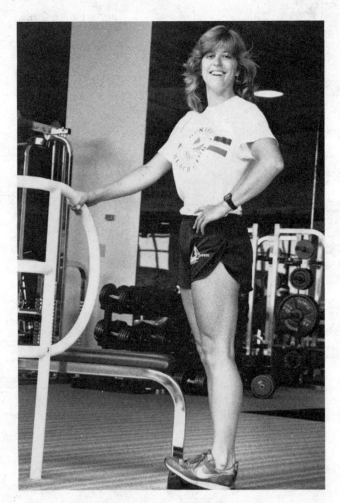

Repeat Exercise #1 two more times.

(The above routine can simply be referred to as "3 sets of Toe Raises 15 reps.)

Exercise #2. Flat-footed Squats — take a broom handle or empty barbell and place it across your shoulders but far enough down that it doesn't touch your neck. Place your feet about shoulder width apart and point them outward. With your back

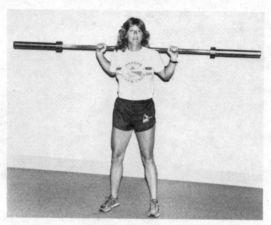

absolutely straight, squat down to a sitting position (while breathing in), stop momentarily (do not bounce!), and then raise yourself back up to a standing position (while breathing out).

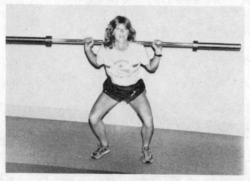

Perform this motion 6 times. As you go on to heavier weights, or, if you are already using heavier weights, it will be necessary to place your barbell on a squat rack and load the weights on there. You will then load the barbell and the weights on your back from the rack and proceed through the squat exercise. Take up to 45 seconds for recovery.

Repeat Exercise #2 two more times.

Exercise #3. Leg Curls — lie down face down on a leg curl bench and put the rear of your ankle underneath the leg curl cushions.

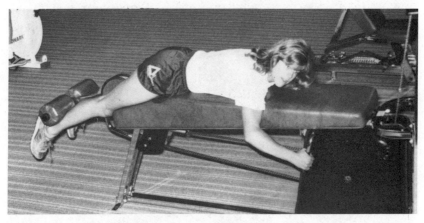

Lift up on the cushions slowly (while breathing out) by bending your legs until you can feel the cushions touch against the back of your thighs.

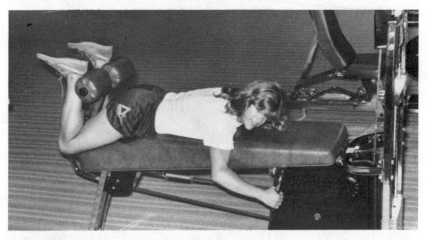

Slowly let the cushion back down (while breathing in). One cycle up and down should take about three seconds.

Perform this motion 6 times but don't allow the weight to rest until you have completed your 6 leg curls. Take up to 45 seconds for recovery.

Repeat Exercise #3 two more times.

Exercise #4. Hyperextensions — position your waist over the front of the front pad of the hyperextension bench. Secure your ankles underneath the back pad of the hyperextension bench. Allow the upper part of your body to assume a position approximately perpendicular to the floor.

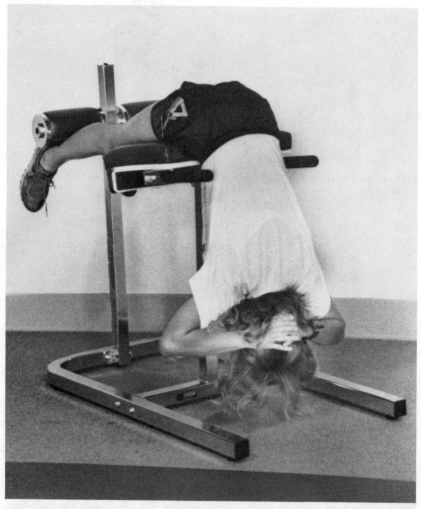

With hands across your chest or behind your neck, attempt to raise (do not swing) your upper body as high as you can (while breathing out).

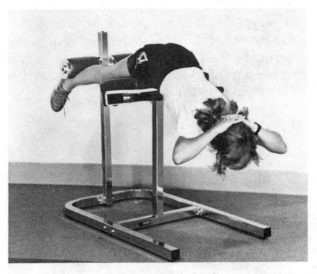

You should at least raise your upper body to a position parallel to the floor.

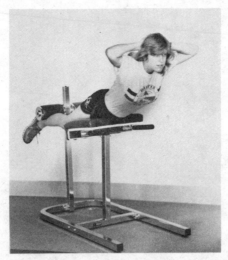

Then allow the upper part of your body to assume a position perpendicular to the floor again (while breathing in). Take at least 2 seconds for one complete cycle. Do as many as you can up to 10. If you can't do one, use your hands to help you. Take up to 30 seconds for recovery.

Repeat Exercise #4 two more times.

Exercise #5. Lat Pulldown — place hands on the lat machine bar about shoulder width apart.

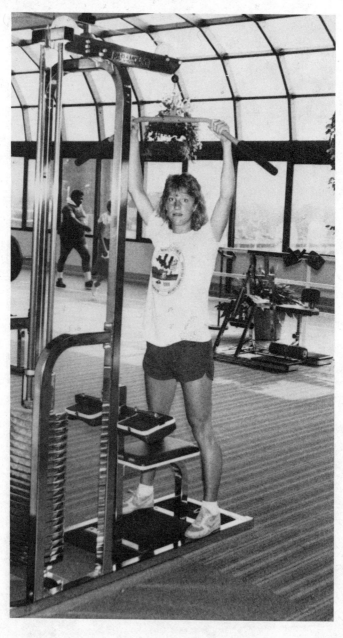

Holding hands straight up in the air, pull the lat machine bar down as you sit down.

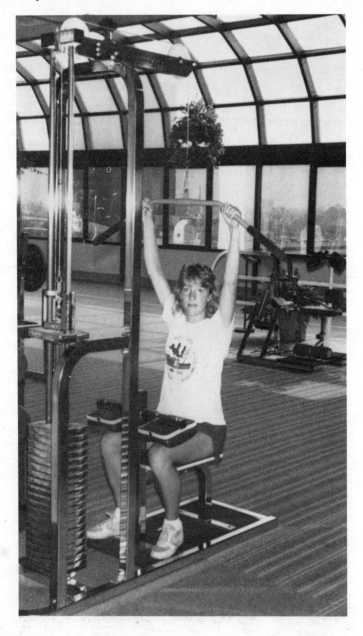

From this position, pull the lat bar down to your chest (while breathing out), keeping your forearms perpendicular to the floor. Allow your arms to straighten out again (while breathing in). One full cycle should take about 2-3 seconds.

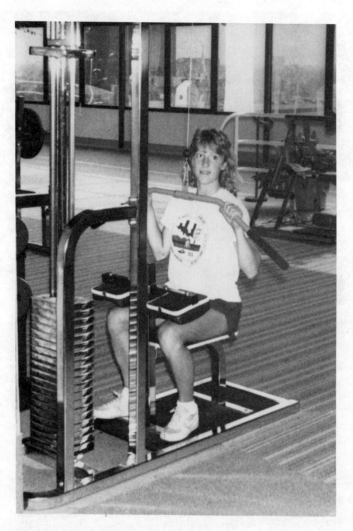

Perform this motion 8 times. Take up to 30 seconds for recovery. Repeat Exercise #5 two more times.

Exercise #6. Dumbell Bent Rows — leaning on something about table height with one hand, assume a position as if you were going to start a gasoline mower by pulling straight up on a cord with the other hand. In the 'cord' hand, place a dumbell.

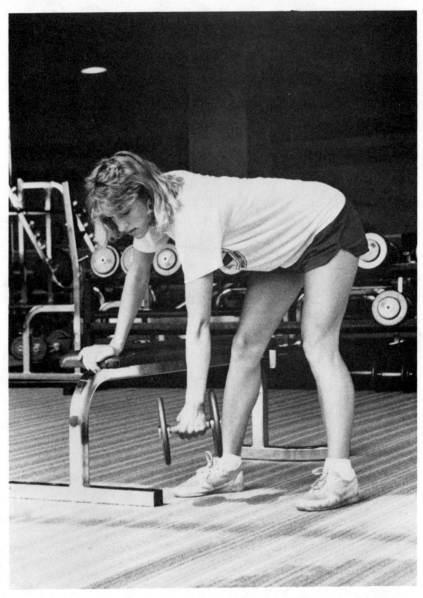

Pull the dumbell straight up to the shoulder (while breathing out) and return it to the original position (while breathing in).

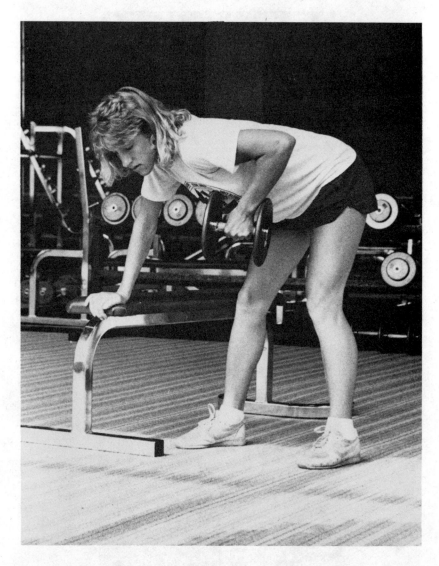

Perform this motion 6 times. Then, perform this motion 6 times with your other hand.

Repeat Exercise #6 two more times.

Exercise #7. Shoulder Shrugs — bend over, pick up a barbell, and assume an upright position.

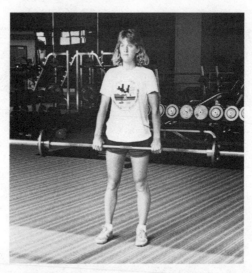

With arms straight, shrug shoulders as far up as possible. Then relax your shoulders. Repeat this exercise 6 times. Return barbell to the floor. Take up to 30 seconds for recovery.

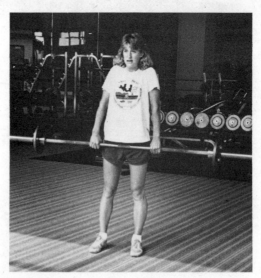

Repeat Exercise #7 two more times.

Exercise #8. Bench Press — lie down on your back on a bench-press bench with your head between the uprights supporting the barbell. Grab the barbell with hands about shoulder width or a little more apart. Lift the barbell off the uprights . . .

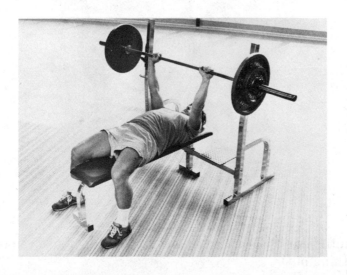

. . . and bring it down to your chest (while breathing in). Make a momentary stop (don't bounce) and then . . .

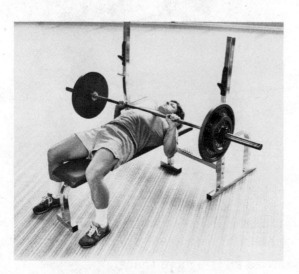

. . . lift it up . . .

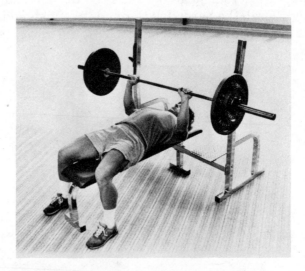

. . . until your arms are extended straight up above you (while breathing out).

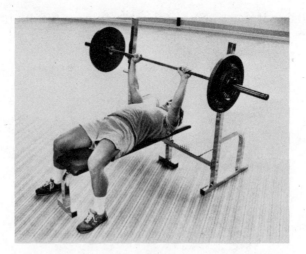

Perform this motion 6 times. On your last lift, return the barbell to the uprights. Take up to 45 seconds for recovery.

Repeat Exercise #8 two more times.

Exercise #9. Pectoral Flyes — grab a dumbell in each hand, sit on a regular weight bench, and lie back, putting your arms straight above you with your palms facing each other.

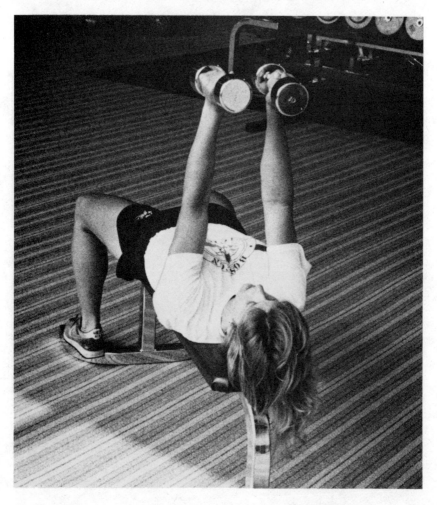

Keeping your arms as straight as possible (they will naturally tend to bend slightly), lower the dumbells sideways (while breathing in) until your arms are parallel to the floor.

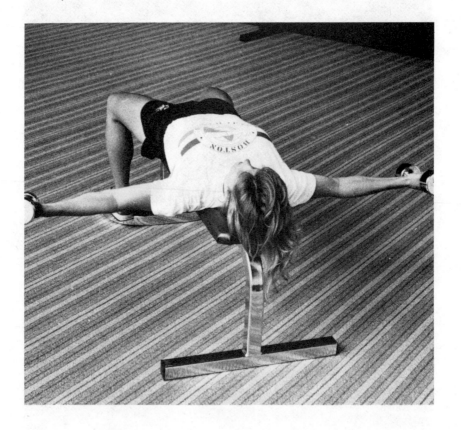

Then raise the dumbells back to the original position (while breathing out). Perform this motion 6 times. Take up to 30 seconds for recovery.

Repeat Exercise #9 two more times.

Exercise #10. Military Press — place an empty barbell on a shoulder-high weight rack and add any weights you are going to use at this time. Facing the barbell, grab it with your hands about shoulder length apart, lift it onto your chest . . .

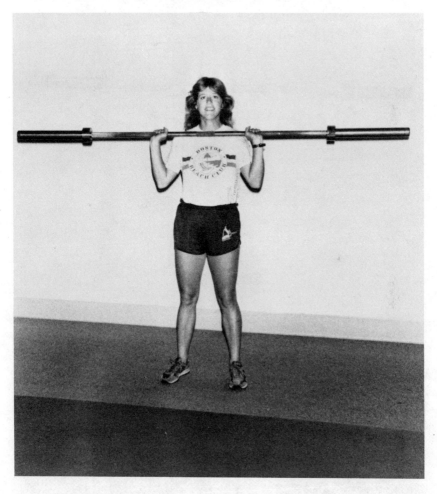

. . . and lift it till your arms are extended above your head (breathing out as you do). Next, lower the barbell to your chest (while breathing in). Do not bounce the barbell on your chest!

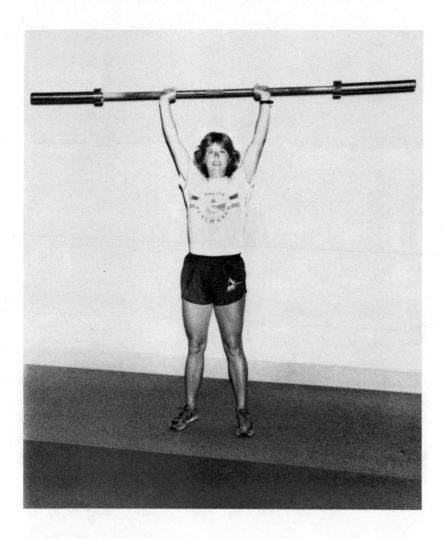

Perform this motion 6 times. Take up to 45 seconds for recovery. Repeat Exercise #10 two more times.

Exercise #11. Side Lateral Raise — pick up two dumbells and hold them to your sides, palms facing in.

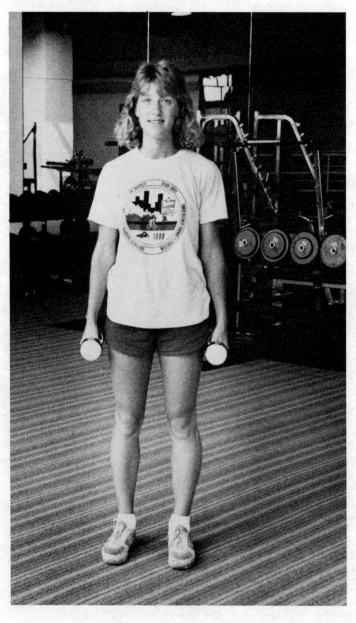

While breathing out, slowly raise your arms sideways away from your body . . .

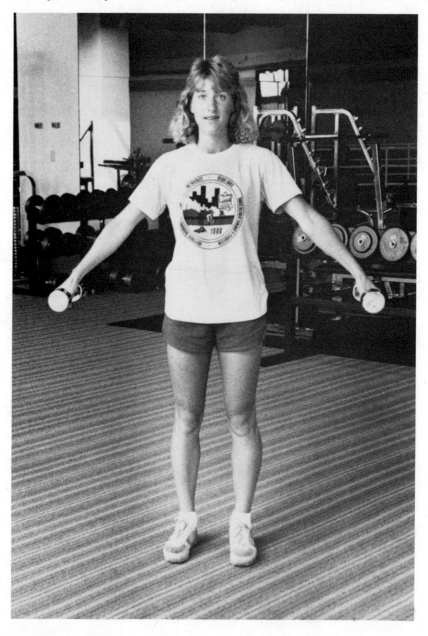

. . . until your arms are parallel to the floor. Hold momentarily and slowly bring your arms back to their original position.

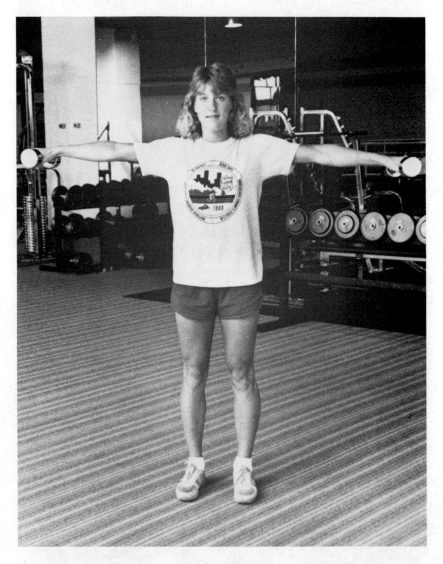

Perform this motion 6 times. Take up to 45 seconds for recovery. Repeat Exercise #11 two more times.

Exercise #12. Curls — pick a barbell or preferably a curling bar
off the floor with palms facing away from you. Standing with
back as straight as possible with bar against your thighs,

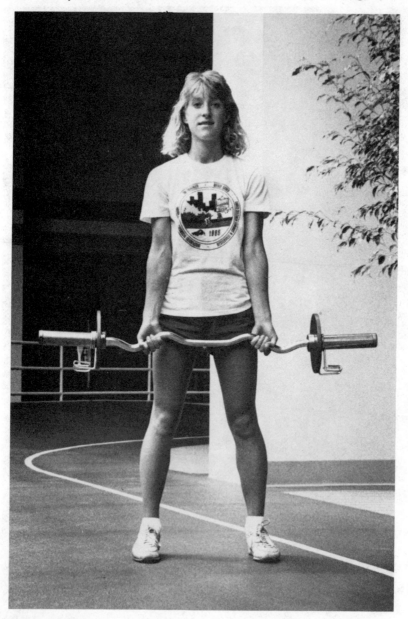

... slowly bend your arms ...

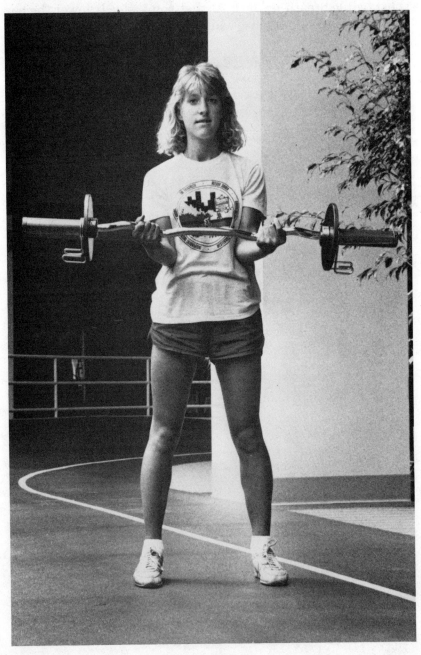

. . . until you have raised the bar in a semicircular motion to your chest (while breathing out). At that point, slowly lower the bar back down to your thighs (while breathing in).

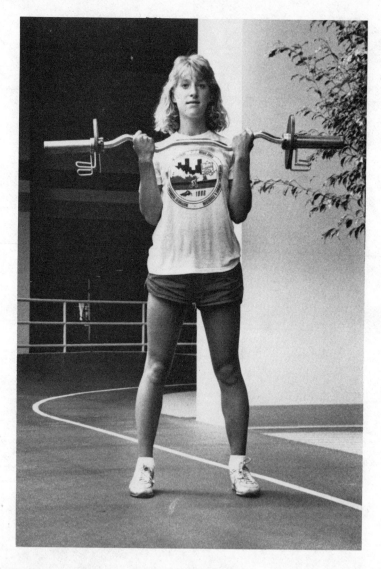

Perform this motion 6 times. Take up to 45 seconds for recovery. Repeat Exercise #12 two more times.

Exercise #13. Dumbell Triceps Extension — stand a dumbell on its side. With palms facing upward, grip the dumbell with both hands so that your palms are placed directly against the underside of the upper bulge and so that your fingers and thumbs tightly encircle the dumbell handle.

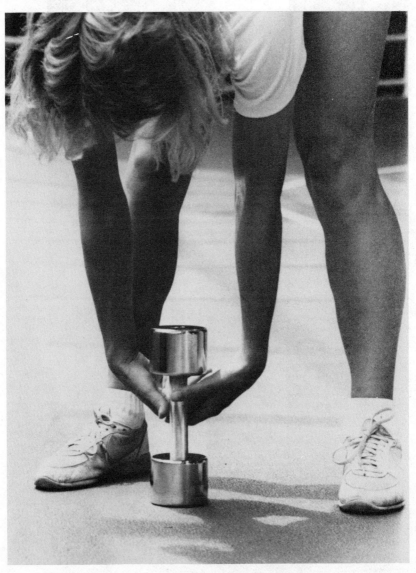

Lift the dumbell carefully over your head. Starting from this position, . . .

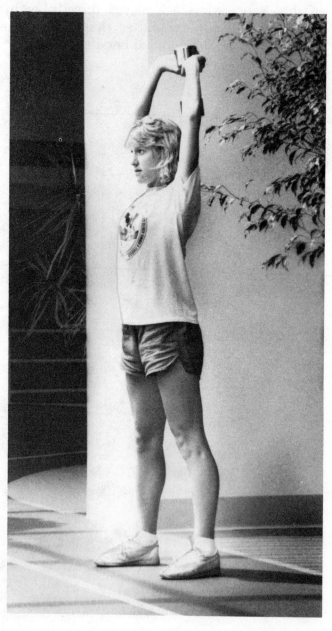

. . . lower the dumbell down behind your head as far as you are able by bending your arms (while breathing in). Next, extend your arms to return the dumbell to the starting position (while breathing out).

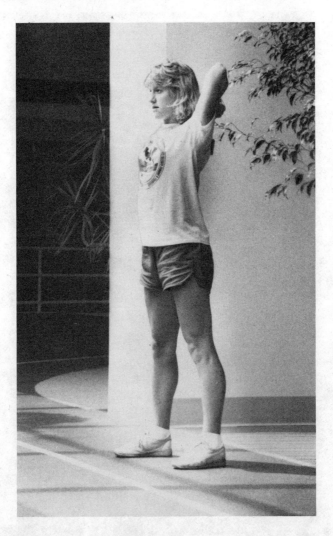

Perform this motion 6 times. Take up to 30 seconds for recovery.

Repeat Exercise #13 two more times.

Exercise #14. Wrist Curl — grab a dumbell with your palm up. Resting your forearm on a weight bench with your wrist over the side, bend your wrist back towards the floor as far as you can. Starting from this position, . . .

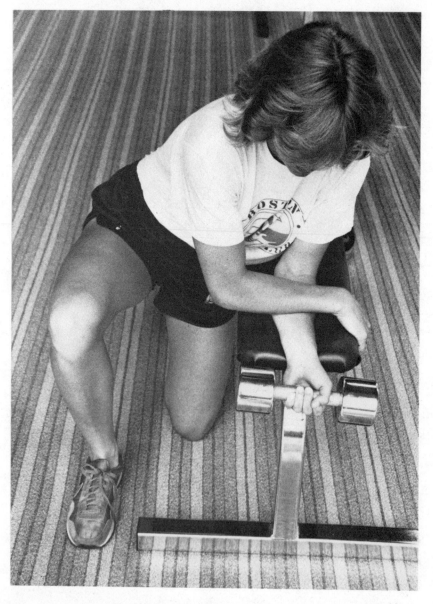

. . . bend your wrist to raise the dumbell as far up as you can without moving your arm. Slowly return the dumbell to the original position. Perform this motion 10 times. Take up to 30 seconds for recovery.

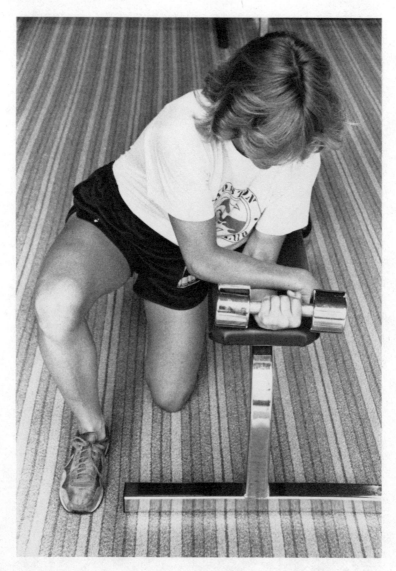

Repeat Exercise #14 two more times.

Exercise #15. Reverse Wrist Curl — grab a dumbell with your palm down. Resting your forearm on a weight bench with your wrist over the side, bend your wrist forward towards the floor as far as you can. Starting from this position, . . .

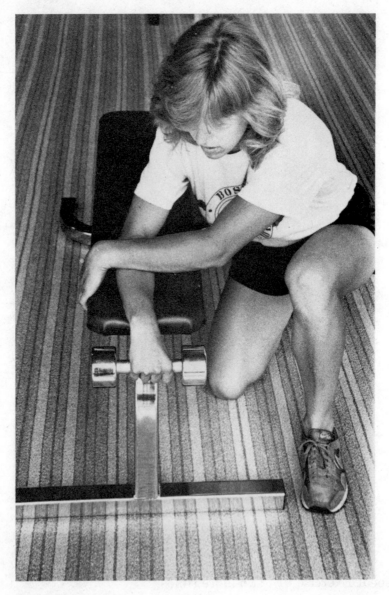

. . . bend you wrist back to raise the dumbell as far up as you can without moving your arm. Slowly return the dumbell to the original position. Perform this motion 10 times. Take up to 30 seconds for recovery.

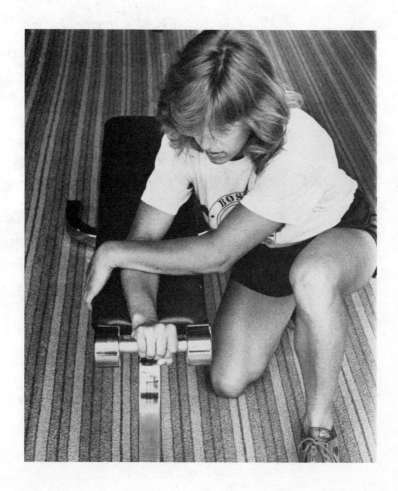

Repeat Exercise #15 two more times.

Exercise #16. Situps — lie down on a situp bench on your back and place your feet under the foot strap or foot bar. With your legs slightly bent and your arms folded across your chest or behind your neck, . . .

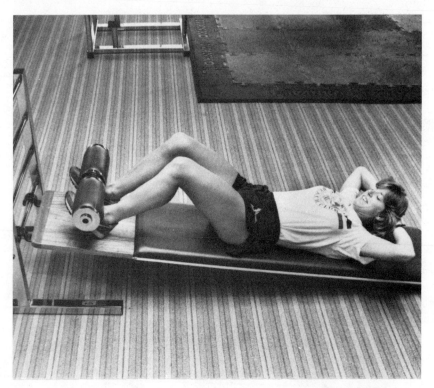

. . . raise your upper body as far forward as you can (while breathing out).

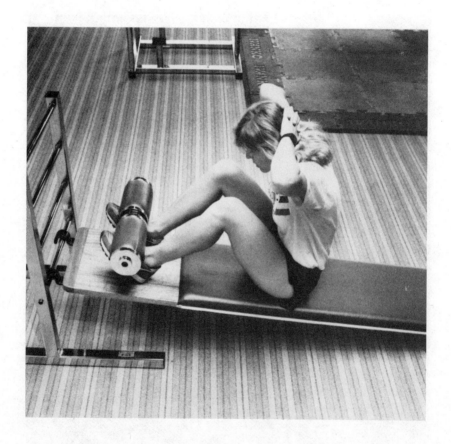

Then slowly lower your upper body till it barely touches the bench (while breathing in). Perform this motion as many times as you can up to 25 times. In the unlikely event that you have trouble doing one situp, raise the head side of the situp bench above the level of the foot straps and proceed doing your situps. Take up to 30 seconds for recovery.

Repeat Exercise #16 two more times.

Exercise #17. Seated Twists — with a broom handle or empty barbell across the back of your shoulders, sit down on a weight bench in a straddle position. Place your hands as far out to each side of the bar as you can.

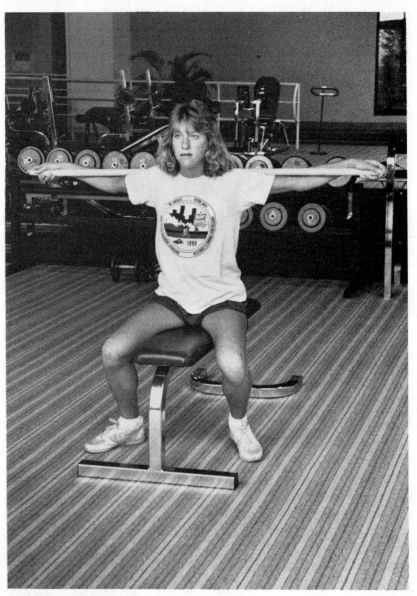

Keeping your hips and legs straight, twist your shoulders and upper body as far to the left as you possibly can.

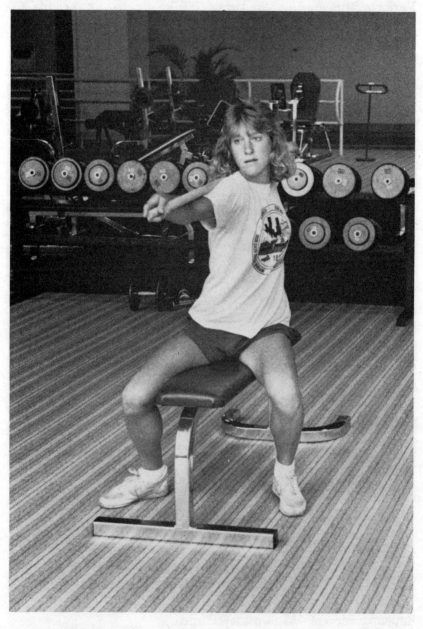

Starting from this position, twist your body as far to the right as you possibly can. Then twist back to the starting position. Perform this motion 25 times. Take up to 30 seconds for recovery.

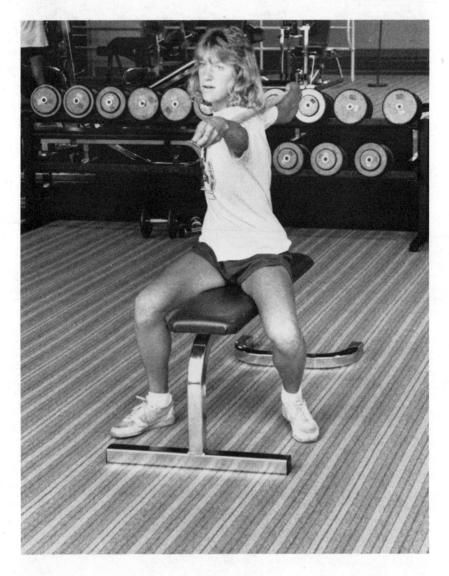

Repeat Exercise #17 two more times.

Exercise #18. Side Bends — with a broom handle or empty barbell across the back of your shoulders, assume a standing position. Place your hands as far out to each side of the bar as you can.

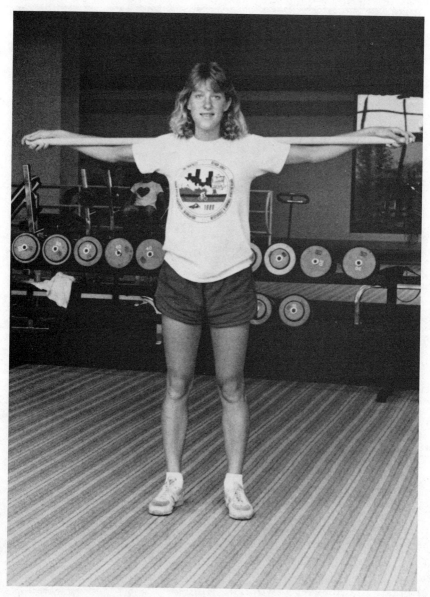

Bend sideways to the left as far as you can. Starting from this position, bend sideways to the the right as far as you can. Then bend your body sideways to the original position. Perform this motion 25 times. Take up to 30 seconds for recovery.

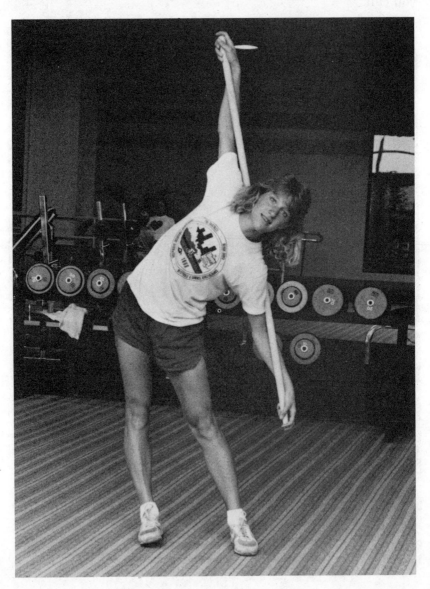

Repeat Exercise #18 two more times.

During your recovery periods, it is often helpful to stretch out by placing your feet shoulder width apart and pointed forward, bending down as far as you can, trying to touch your hands or your palms as close to the floor as you can without feeling pain, and resting in that position until your next exercise. Another simple stretch you might find helpful during the recovery periods can be done by kneeling down on the floor, pointing your toes to the rear, and sitting down on your heels until your next exercise. Still another maneuver you might find helpful is the following. With your left foot three feet in front of your right, bend the knee of your front foot while keeping your right leg straight and your right foot flat on the ground until you feel your calf stretching. Hold this position for about 5 seconds. Then perform this maneuver starting with your right foot in front of your left.

During these recovery periods, you should feel free to use any other maneuver that you feel will help you perform the next task. However remember that maneuvers done during recovery should take very little energy since the main purpose of the recovery periods is to rest. Many times, you may need your recovery time for total rest — both physical and mental. Take it. Listen to your body and let it guide you.

How to determine the amount of weight to use

If you are experienced with weight-lifting and are familiar with the amount of weight you can handle with each of the exercises in the Basic Exercise Program, you can begin the above schedule right away. However, if you've never been on a weight-lifting program before, you should use the following four sessions to develop form and to help you determine the amount of weight you should use on each of the exercises of the basic program.

These sessions should be done at a health club or spa, preferably under the watchful eye of an employee of the spa. This person should give you useful pointers as to your form. He or she should also be able to "spot" you, that is, to catch you if you lose balance or are unable to control the weight you are lifting. If you are in the rare situation where you do not have access to a health club or spa, have someone available to spot you.

You should allow yourself a day off between these initial sessions. If you start out on a Monday for example, you should have sessions on Monday, Wednesday, Friday, and finish your fourth session on the following Monday.

The following chart outlines the first of these four sessions. In the first column of this chart are the numbers of the exercises from the Basic Exercise Program as described above. In the second column are the values representing the weight you should begin with for each exercise. In the third column is the number of times you should *try* to perform that exercise (referred to as the number of attempted reps). The fourth column is blank and you should use it to record the number of times you were able to do that particular exercise using the recommended weight (the number of reps you actually completed). Remember, the most important thing you can do as you are going through these sessions is to develop proper form and coordination. *Don't sacrifice your form to do one more rep.* Try as hard as you please but don't do it at the expense of your form.

As you get done with each exercise, write down the number of reps you did in column 4 in the table below. *Do only one set of each exercise.* That is, once you have done as many reps as you can up to 25 reps without stopping, don't try to do the exercise over again. Just go on to the next exercise. You can take as long as one full minute of rest between each exercise during these four sessions.

First Session

Exercise	Weight to use	Reps attempted (pounds)	Reps completed
#1	0	25	_____
#2	0*	25	_____
#3	20	25	_____
#4	0	25	_____
#5	20	25	_____
#6	5	25	_____
#7	25•	25	_____
#8	25•	25	_____
#9	5	25	_____
#10	25•	25	_____
#11	3	25	_____
#12	25•	25	_____
#13	5	25	_____
#14	5	25	_____
#15	3	25	_____
#16	0	25	_____
#17	0*	25	_____
#18	0*	25	_____

---

*Use a broom handle for these exercises.
•Use a regular empty (unloaded) barbell for these exercises.

During the first four sessions, exercises #1, #4, #16, #17, and #18 should be done without any weight (except for a broom handle where indicated).

If you are not successful in doing a particular exercise 25 times, stay at the same weight level for that exercise in you next session. If you are successful in doing 25 reps, increase the weights you use for that exercise according to the following schedule:

Exercise	Pounds
#1	0
#2	0*→25•→50→80
#3	20→30→50→80
#4	0
#5	20→30→50→80
#6	5→10→20→40
#7	25•→35→55→85
#8	25•→35→55→85
#9	5→10→20→40
#10	25•→35→55→85
#11	3→5→10→20
#12	25•→35→55→85
#13	5→10→20→40
#14	5→10→20→40
#15	3→5→10→20
#16	0
#17	0*
#18	0*

---

*Use a broom handle for these exercises.
•Use a regular empty (unloaded) barbell for these exercises.

Thus, for example, if you are able to do 25 reps of exercise #10 in the first session, increase the weight you use from 25 pounds (an unloaded barbell) to 35 pounds. In the second session, if you are not able to do 25 reps at 35 pounds, use 35 pounds again for the third session. If during the third session, you are able to do 25 reps at 35 pounds, increase the weights you use to 55 pounds for use in the fourth and final of the initial sessions. Be sure to record the number of reps performed and the amount of weight you used for each session on the following forms.

Second Session

Exercise	Weight used (pounds)	Reps attempted	Reps completed
#1	_0_	25	____
#2	_____	25	____
#3	_____	25	____
#4	_0_	25	____
#5	_____	25	____
#6	_____	25	____
#7	_____	25	____
#8	_____	25	____
#9	_____	25	____
#10	_____	25	____
#11	_____	25	____
#12	_____	25	____
#13	_____	25	____
#14	_____	25	____
#15	_____	25	____
#16	_0_	25	____
#17	_0_	25	____
#18	_0_	25	____

Third Session

Exercise	Weight used (pounds)	Reps attempted	Reps completed
#1	__0__	25	_____
#2	_____	25	_____
#3	_____	25	_____
#4	__0__	25	_____
#5	_____	25	_____
#6	_____	25	_____
#7	_____	25	_____
#8	_____	25	_____
#9	_____	25	_____
#10	_____	25	_____
#11	_____	25	_____
#12	_____	25	_____
#13	_____	25	_____
#14	_____	25	_____
#15	_____	25	_____
#16	__0__	25	_____
#17	__0__	25	_____
#18	__0__	25	_____

Fourth Session

Exercise	Weight used (pounds)	Reps attempted	Reps completed
#1	__0__	25	____
#2	_____	25	____
#3	_____	25	____
#4	__0__	25	____
#5	_____	25	____
#6	_____	25	____
#7	_____	25	____
#8	_____	25	____
#9	_____	25	____
#10	_____	25	____
#11	_____	25	____
#12	_____	25	____
#13	_____	25	____
#14	_____	25	____
#15	_____	25	____
#16	__0__	25	____
#17	__0__	25	____
#18	__0__	25	____

Let us assume that you have completed the initial four sessions
and you have recorded the pounds used and the reps you
completed for each of the 18 exercises. The above table would
be filled out and look something like the following:

Fourth Session

Exercise	Weight used (pounds)	Reps attempted	Reps completed
#1	_0_	25	_25_
#2	_50_	25	_22_
#3	_30_	25	_24_
#4	_0_	25	_12_
#5	_50_	25	_3_
#6	_10_	25	_21_
#7	_55_	25	_18_
#8	_85_	25	_12_
#9	_10_	25	_10_
#10	_55_	25	_8_
#11	_5_	25	_15_
#12	_35_	25	_22_
#13	_20_	25	_14_
#14	_10_	25	_25_
#15	_5_	25	_25_
#16	_0_	25	_21_
#17	_0_	25	_25_
#18	_0_	25	_25_

Using these results along with the following table, you can
determine the amount of weight you should use for your first
regular session.

Weight Used (pounds)

Number of Reps	3	5	10	20	25	30	35	40	50	55	80	85
1	3	5	10	15	25	30	30	30	40	45	65	70
2	3	5	10	15	25	30	30	30	40	45	65	70
3	3	5	10	15	25	30	30	30	40	45	70	75
4	3	5	10	15	25	30	30	35	40	50	70	75
5	3	5	10	15	25	30	30	35	40	50	75	80
6	3	5	10	20	25	30	30	35	45	50	75	80
7	3	5	10	20	25	30	30	35	50	55	80	85
8	3	5	10	20	25	30	35	40	50	55	80	85
9	3	5	10	20	25	30	35	40	50	55	85	90
10	3	5	10	20	25	30	35	40	55	60	85	90
11	3	5	10	20	25	30	40	45	55	60	90	95
12	3	5	10	20	30	35	40	45	55	60	90	95
13	3	5	10	25	30	35	40	45	60	65	95	100
14	3	5	15	25	30	35	40	50	60	65	95	100
15	3	5	15	25	30	35	40	50	60	65	100	105
16	3	5	15	25	30	35	40	50	65	70	100	105
17	3	10	15	25	30	35	40	55	65	70	105	110
18	5	10	15	25	30	35	40	55	65	70	105	110
19	5	10	15	25	30	40	45	55	70	75	110	115
20	5	10	15	25	30	40	45	60	70	75	110	115
21	5	10	15	25	35	40	45	60	70	75	115	120
22	5	10	15	25	35	40	45	60	75	80	115	120
23	5	10	15	30	35	40	45	65	75	80	120	125
24	5	10	15	30	35	40	45	65	75	80	120	125
25	5	10	15	30	35	40	45	65	80	85	125	130

For example, since you have done exercise #1 without any
weight, you will use no weight in your first regular workout (the
Basic Exercise Program). On your chart, you find that you have
done 22 reps of exercise #2 (squats) using 50 pounds of weight.
Referring to the table, you find that you will be able to start your
exercise #2 using 75 pounds of weight. Similarly, you should
use the above table and your chart to determine the weights for
each of the exercises and write them down.

Using the chart and table above, we can produce the following
schedule:

Exercise Number	Weight to Use for the First Regular Session
#1	0
#2	75 pounds
#3	45 pounds
#4	0
#5	40 pounds
#6	15 pounds
#7	70 pounds
#8	95 pounds
#9	10 pounds
#10	55 pounds
#11	5 pounds
#12	45 pounds
#13	25 pounds
#14	15 pounds
#15	10 pounds
#16	0
#17	0
#18	0

Now, using the chart from your fourth session, fill out the following form to determine the weights you should use for your first regular session.

Exercise Number	Weight to Use for the First Regular Session
#1	0
#2	____ pounds
#3	____ pounds
#4	0
#5	____ pounds
#6	____ pounds
#7	____ pounds
#8	____ pounds
#9	____ pounds
#10	____ pounds
#11	____ pounds
#12	____ pounds
#13	____ pounds
#14	____ pounds
#15	____ pounds
#16	0
#17	0
#18	0

When you do your first regular session on the Basic Exercise Program, you should again have a health club employee or friend watch you. The routine should go quite easily and from that point on you should be able to make it pretty much on your own. However, aside from the extra margin of safety afforded by having someone there to help you, it is extremely worthwhile for you to find a friend who will go on the program with you. Having someone go on the program with you makes your program more of a social event. You can use each other for mutual motivation. Two people going through a workout together is also time efficient. While one person is doing the exercise, the other is resting and spotting.

I recommend that you stay with the weights that you start the Basic Exercise Program with for at least one to two weeks so you begin to get used to the routine. At that time, try to increase the weights you use in each exercise by 5 pounds each session. When you find you are straining too hard to do six repetitions, pull back 5 pounds and try to increase your number of reps until you reach ten. Then add 5 pounds and continue to work your way up from there.

Pain

Pain is your body's way of telling you where you are. Besides all the other objections I have regarding the harmful effects of drugs, I must especially urge you to stay away from pain killers and narcotic drugs. Going on an exercise program with pain killing drugs is like flying a jet plane with a blindfold. As you exercise, you must be acutely aware of your body. As you start out on the program from a previously inactive life-style, you will experience pain, not so much on the days you do the exercises as you will on the following day. For many, this is all the excuse they need to give up. However, this experience of pain is necessary for you to be able to monitor your body. As your activity levels and your nutrition improve, the pain you experience will tend to go away.

Pain lets you know that the bones in your body are rejuvenating themselves. It lets you know that you are turning over old muscle tissue and are adding muscle mass. The pain of being short of breath is a signal that your body, if provided with the proper nutrients, will increase its oxygen carrying capacity. Pain lets you know that your body is making changes inside and out that will make you feel good and look good.

Pain also serves as a signal to let you know that something is wrong. It is important for you to learn the difference between the "pain of strain" and the "pain of oncoming problems". While I have learned the difference between the two for my own body, it is difficult to put it into words.

I will say however that the pain of strain is much, much, much more common for a person starting the program in reasonably good health. In general, "the pain of strain" is dull, agonizing, and should not persist for more than a few weeks. For example, if you come onto the program with a case of painful "tennis elbow", certain exercises such as curls will seem extremely painful and you might tend to avoid these exercises. However, within a few weeks, it is quite likely that this condition, which may have previously existed for months or years, will go away completely. The same is true with other aches and pains in the body. Physical activity provides the stimulus to get your body to do a general housecleaning, taking care of most and probably all of the problems that it did not have the stimulus or the nutrition to take care of previously.

The pain that warns you of potential oncoming problems is usually sharper. You may feel a sharp pain — a cramp — or you may feel as if a nerve was hit or one of your joints went out. This tells you to stop what your are doing immediately. You may massage the affected area, pull it out, or allow it to rest until your next session. If you feel that your pain is giving you a warning, you might consider calling a sports physician, an osteopathic physician, a chiropractic physician, a mechanotherapist, a massotherapist, or a podiatrist and tell them your problem. After seeing them or talking with them a few times, you will get a better idea of what your various pains are telling you.

More often than pain, light-headedness will be a warning worth listening to. It is due to the fact that because you are using more oxygen and blood sugar to move your body, not enough is making it to your brain and your brain is letting you know that it is beginning to shut down. This tells you to stop what your are doing immediately. After a few minutes, you should be able to begin your routine again. As you keep on the program, your body will adapt to your increased activity levels and this problem will go away. In addition, when you are not engaged in physical activity, you will find that while at rest, you are more alert. This is because the Basic Exercise Program (as well as exercise in general) stimulates your body to become more oxygenated and helps it provide a more abundant food supply to the brain.

Scheduling your sessions

After eating, let at least one hour and preferably two or more hours pass before you begin your workout. Ideally, foods heavy in fat or protein should not be eaten for three hours before you work out. Fruits and vegetables can be reasonably well tolerated up to about one hour before the workout, and water should be supplied in reasonable amounts just before the workout — and during the workout, if necessary. Remember, distilled water is preferable.

If you work regular hours, early in the morning before work (if you are a morning person) or immediately after work provide the two best times for doing your Basic Exercise Program. In both cases, you should eat only after the workout is completed. Fruit with a high water content is probably the best food to have immediately after a workout. Then, after taking a shower, you can eat a regular meal.

Other activities

The Basic Exercise Program is just that — nothing more, nothing less. While it provides you with a highly concentrated form of exercise that will vastly improve your health and performance, there are a number of other activities that not only can improve your health in other ways, but also can help bring joy and excitement to your life and give you a feeling of being *alive*.

Some of these activities are listed on page 141.

While the Basic Exercise Program is a program you can stay on for the rest of your life, after six months to a year on the program, you may consider adding more variety to it. There are a number of books that deal with weight lifting in far greater detail than I have even attempted to deal with here and these books may help you introduce new exercises into your workout. In addition, the manager of a health club might be able to help add more variety to your program. However, if you are a beginner, make sure you stay on the Basic Exercise Program for at least six months before making changes. Sometimes, health club employees let their egos carry them away and they will suggest that their program is better for you than the Basic Exercise Program. Stick with the Basic Exercise Program. While it is not the best program that will ever be devised for beginners, it is better than most of the alternative programs that might be suggested to you by others and guarantees you a standard of quality and safety.

With the nutritional and exercise programs outlined above and environmental health programs outlined in Chapter 8, you can reduce your cancer risk by over 90%, and substantially reduce or eliminate your chances of suffering from degenerative diseases such as osteoporosis, arthritis, and heart disease.

Chapter 7

Tips on Food Preparation

"An important breakthrough occurred in the 1960's when precise and rapid methods for estimating the vitamin, mineral, and amino acid content of raw foods and food products were developed. By the use of those procedures, it was soon proven that significant amounts of nutrients in processed (cooked and stored) foods were reduced, at times seriously . . . "

Robert S. Harris (M.I.T.)

While this book does not pretend to be a cookbook, I think you will find the following tips helpful in preserving as much of the nutritional value of the foods you purchase as possible. In this section, I include guides for substituting safe and more nutritious ingredients for some of the ingredients called for by other recipes or for some of the ingredients that you are currently using.

When you start changing your eating habits, you should make most of your changes gradually.

For example, if you are eating more than 4-8 units of animal protein in your diet per day, try to bring it down within the range of 4-8 units a day (see page 75). Don't try to become a vegetarian overnight. Stay on a 4-8 unit animal protein diet for a few months, or 12 units if you are on an extremely vigorous exercise program. After that time you may consider further reductions or the complete elimination of animal protein from your diet if you wish to become a vegetarian — or you may decide that you feel better with 4-8 units of animal protein in your diet. If in doubt, use the performance tests outlined in Chapter 9 to help you decide how you perform best. Listen to your body.

The same also goes for putting more raw foods into your diet. If you have been eating the average American diet, don't jump into a totally raw foods diet. Slowly work more and more fresh raw foods into your diet and give your body time to adapt.

However, there are some items that you should absolutely remove from your diet immediately. These include all refined sugars and flours, trash fats, and food additives, as well as foods containing them. These foods are listed on the "Foods to Stay Away from Table" in Chapter 5 (page 36). If you are extremely addicted to some of them, do the best that you can. For example, if you feel you would absolutely die if you had to stop eating ice cream, stick with ice creams, such as Haagen Daaz honey vanilla or carob, which are made with honey instead of sugar. Since most ice cream places do not serve these brands, you will find it more difficult to eat ice cream as often, yet you will not have the desperate feeling that you will never be able to eat ice cream again in your life.

Most vegetables should be eaten raw. If you slice vegetables, try to slice them just before serving them. If you juice them, try to juice them just before serving them. Slicing or juicing them way ahead of time will tend to lower their nutritional quality.

Many have gotten used to eating mayonnaises with raw vegetables. While mayonnaises are extremely high in fat, if you must use them, I suggest you use the following recipe or a similar recipe for making your own.

Separate two egg yolks and put them into a blender. To the yolks add

- 2 ounces of water,
- 1 ounce lemon of juice
- 1 teaspoon of salt,
- 1/2 teaspoon of honey (or another natural sweetener),

- 1/2 teaspoon of dry mustard,
- 1/8 teaspoon of cayenne pepper.

Turn blender on low speed and slowly add any bland cold-pressed oil. When the mixture gets too thick to mix, turn the blender on high speed and continue adding oil until thick once more. You should be able to coax in 14-16 ounces of oil.

Similarly, many find that eating vegetable salads is more enjoyable with salad dressing. What follows are some tips on how to create your own gourmet salad dressings.

In the above mayonnaise recipe, replace the water and lemon juice with the following: A mixture containing two ounces of vinegar, one ounce of water, 1-2 cloves of peeled garlic and/or onion, and any combination of spices that pleases you. Blend, then add oil, using only the lower speed on your blender. When this stops blending the mixture properly, you are done.

For an oil and vinegar dressing, you might try the following. Add 2 ounces of vinegar to a measuring cup. Slice and add
- 1/2 medium onion (chopped-up finely),
- 1-2 medium sized cloves of garlic (minced),
- 1/2 teaspoon of oregano, and
- salt and pepper to taste.
Stir and then add 3-4 ounces of olive oil (or the cold-pressed oil of your choice). Shake before using or toss into a salad.

Some vegetables, such as potato, sweet potato, yams, squashes, corn (in the husk) can be baked in the oven at 350 degrees for 45-75 minutes. The mild steaming of vegetables (such as spinach, broccoli, sliced cabbage, sliced onion, sliced carrots, beet greens, cauliflower, asparagus, dandelion greens, Brussels sprouts, sliced kohlrabi, sliced squash, green beans, yellow beans, peas, sliced turnips, sliced rutabagas, sliced beets, sliced parsnips, artichokes, sliced eggplant, sliced potatoes, corn (husked), sliced sweetpotato, and sliced yams) improves their edibility and may give them added flavor. When steaming, try to keep a slight amount of crunch to the vegetable, or if you insist on getting rid of all the crunchiness, stop cooking the vegetable as soon as the crunchiness is out.

When steaming, use enough water to make sure that the steamer does not go dry but no more than a cup. Steamers can be purchased at culinary supply shops as well as some department stores, food stores, and discount stores. Vegetables that are thick should be sliced to insure uniform cooking and to prevent overcooking during the steaming process. Steamed vegetables may be eaten plain or with butter or oil, salt and spices.

If you decide to fry your vegetables, use either cold pressed peanut oil, olive oil, sesame oil, or butter. Using a skillet or wok, add the oil before heating the pan. Then preheat the oil until the addition of a drop of water to the oil in the pan produces a sizzle. (Butter will sizzle on its own since it contains water.) Then add the vegetable, whole (if it is small), sliced, or diced. Cook it for as short a time as possible. Again, it doesn't hurt to retain a little crunchiness to the vegetable or vegetable combination. Frying provides the opportunity for you to add dry and fresh spices during the cooking process. Fresh garlic, onions, parsley, dill and other fresh spices, sauteed in with your vegetables (and/ or meat) will impart a variety of flavors to the foods you prepare.

Vegetables cooked as described above will generally have better vitamin retentions than those indicated in the following table.

Retention of Vitamins of Various Cooked Vegetables

Food	Vit. C	Vit. B1	Vit. B2	Vit. B3	Vit. B5	Vit. B6	Vit. Bc	Vit. A.
Baked Potato	80%	85%	95%	95%	90%	95%	90%	
Boiled Potato (with skin)	75%	80%	95%	95%	90%	95%	90%	
Boiled Potato (without skin)	75%	80%	95%	95%	90%	95%	75%	
Fried Potato	80%	80%	95%	95%	90%	95%	75%	
Baked Sweetpotato	80%	85%	95%	95%	90%	95%	90%	90%
Boiled Sweetpotato	75%	80%	95%	95%	90%	95%	90%	85%
Tomatoes,baked or boiled	95%	95%	95%	95%	95%	95%	70%	95%
Boiled Dark Leafy Greens (e.g. beet greens, Chinese cabbage, collards, kale, mustard greens, spinach, swiss chard, turnip greens)	60%	85%	95%	90%	95%	90%	65%	95%
Boiled Roots, Bulbs, Squash, and Fresh (immature) Beans (e.g. carrots, beets, green peas, onions, parsnips, rutabaga, squash, sweet corn, turnips, fresh beans in pods)	70%	85%	95%	95%	90%	95%	70%	90%
Other Boiled Vegetables (e.g. asparagus, bean sprouts, broccoli, Brussels sprouts, cabbage, cauliflower, eggplant, okra, sweet peppers)	80%	85%	95%	90%	90%	90%	70%	90%

All fruits should be eaten raw. If you slice fruits, try to slice them just before serving them. If you juice them, try to juice them just before serving them. Slicing or juicing them way ahead of time will tend to lower their nutritional quality.

When making fruit salads, try to avoid adding any sweeteners. If you must, sweeten the salad with apple juice or frozen concentrated fruit juices that contain no added sugar.

Making juices from fresh fruits results in a change in the nutrient composition. In general, it is best to eat fruits whole rather than juiced. However, as can be seen below, some vitamin and mineral contents are enriched in the juice as compared to the whole fruit. Juices also provide you with the opportunity of getting more nutrients into your body. Most people, for example could not get as much vitamin A or as much vitamin C from eating whole carrots or oranges as they could from drinking juices made from them. In cases where an increased vitamin intake is necessary, juices are certainly preferable to vitamin pills. Juices also serve as a suitable alternative to soft drinks.

Nutrient Content of Fruits and Fresh Juices*

Food	Calcium	Iron	Man-ganese	Vit. C	Vit. B1	Vit. B2	Vit. B3	Vit. B5	Vit. B6	Vit. Bc
Grapefruit	0.30	0.10	0.10	16.82	0.75	0.36	0.43	1.56	0.59	0.7
Grapefruit Juice	0.19	0.28	0.13	16.24	0.68	0.30	0.27	0.88	0.51	0.6
Lemon	0.75	1.15	0.26	30.46	0.92	0.41	0.18	1.19	1.25	0.9
Lemon Juice	0.23	0.07	0.08	30.67	0.80	0.24	0.21	0.75	0.93	1.2
Lime	0.92	1.11	0.07	16.17	0.67	0.39	0.35	1.32	0.65	0.6
Lime Juice	0.28	0.06	0.07	18.09	0.49	0.22	0.19	0.93	0.72	0.7
Orange	0.71	0.12	0.13	18.87	1.23	0.50	0.32	0.97	0.58	1.6
Orange Juice	0.20	0.25	0.08	18.52	1.33	0.39	0.47	0.77	0.40	1.6
Tangerine	0.27	0.13	0.18	11.67	1.59	0.29	0.19	0.83	0.69	1.1
Tangerine Juice	0.35	0.26	0.22	12.02	0.93	0.27	0.12	0.53	0.44	0.2

*Units in this table are given in terms of RDAs per1000 calories

Nuts and seeds should be eaten raw. While their occasional use in bakery products is all right, whenever you purchase them or eat them by themselves, they should be eaten raw so that you can avoid the loss of nutritional value that occurs when they are roasted.

Vitamin Loss During Processing of Dry Nuts and Seeds
(RDAs per 1000 Calories)

Food	Vitamin B1
Almonds Dried	0.24
Almonds Dried Blanched	0.18
Almonds Toasted	0.15
Almonds Dry Roasted	0.15
Almonds Oil Roasted	0.14
Almond Butter	0.14
Almonds Oil Roasted/blanched	0.08
Filberts Dried	0.53
Filbert Dried Blanched	0.51
Filberts Oil Roasted	0.22
Filberts Dry Roasted	0.21
Macadamia Nuts Dried	0.33
Macadamia Oil Roasted	0.20
Peanuts Dried	0.78
Peanuts Oil Roasted	0.34
Peanut Butter	0.17
Pecans Dried	0.85
Pecans Dry Roasted	0.32
Pecans Oil Roasted	0.30
Pistachio Nuts Dried	0.95
Pistachio Dry Roasted	0.47
Sunflower Seeds Dried	2.68
Sunflower Seed Butter	0.37
Sunflower Seed Toasted	0.35
Sunflower Seed Oil Roasted	0.35
Sunflower Seed Dry Roasted	0.12

In western diets, oysters and clams are the only raw meats that are consumed to any considerable extent. Sushi bars (where fish is served raw) have become popular in certain cosmopolitan areas. In some gourmet restaurants, beef tartar (ground beef served raw with herbs and spices) is served. However in general, the use of raw meats in the United States has not and probably will not be accepted widely in the foreseeable future.

What is important for those who do eat it is that *meat should be cooked as little as possible.* For red meats, that means eating meat as rare as possible. For fish, chicken, and pork, it means *not* cooking the meat until they become dried out, but rather cooking them so that they still retain a significant amount of moisture. In general, broiling or roasting meat for as short a time as possible preserves the greatest amount of nutrition. Lightly sauteeing organs (such as liver, kidney, and heart) in olive oil or butter is the most convenient way to preserve their very high nutritional quality. Many people who have an aversion to eating liver develop this aversion because of the grainy texture of liver that comes when liver is overcooked.

Meats cooked as described above will generally have better vitamin retentions than those indicated in the table below.

Vitamin Retention during the Cooking of Meat

	Vit. B1	Vit. B2	Vit. B3	Vit. B5	Vit. B6	Vit. Bc
CHICKEN MEAT						
Fried	63%	76%	64%	60%	61%	54%
Roasted	59%	79%	70%	65%	68%	54%
Stewed	45%	77%	50%	47%	41%	58%
BEEF						
Broiled	70%	92%	78%	79%	74%	87%
Roasted	58%	98%	75%	97%	66%	88%
Braised (stewed)	45%	86%	61%	69%	46%	74%
PORK						
Broiled	70%	100%	80%	80%	80%	
Roasted	60%	95%	85%	60%	85%	
Braised (stewed)	40%	75%	80%	55%	70%	
FISH (Baked or Broiled)	90-95%	95-100%	95-100%			

The nutritional quality of eggs is best preserved when the egg is cooked as gently as possible without breaking the shell or the yolk. Thus a soft boiled egg is preferable to a lightly fried egg, but a fried egg is preferable to a scrambled egg. Similarly, a soft boiled egg is preferable to a hard boiled egg.

Vitamin Values* for Eggs Prepared in Various Ways

FOOD	Iron	Vit. A	Vit. B1	Vit. B2	Vit. B5	Vit. B6	Vit. Bc	Vit. B1
CHICKEN EGG								
Raw	0.74	0.99	0.37	1.12	1.99	0.35	1.03	3.2
Hard-boiled**	0.74	0.99	0.31	1.07	1.99	0.33	0.78	2.7
Poached	0.73	0.99	0.29	0.95	1.99	0.29	0.78	2.6
Fried	0.62	1.00	0.26	0.90	1.67	0.27	0.65	2.3
Omelet Or Scrambled	0.55	0.94	0.28	0.97	1.58	0.28	0.59	2.2

*Values given in terms of RDAs per 1000 calories.
**Soft boiled eggs will have a vitamin level between those for raw and those for hard-boiled.

Dry beans and grains, while excellent whole foods, are virtually inedible unless they are processed. The easiest way to process them is to soak them in water overnight. Beans and grains which have been soaked overnight should be drained, rinsed, and drained again. At this point you can do one of two things with them: (1) sprout them or (2) cook them.

Sprouting

Sprouting is simple and is the only form of food processing that actually increases food value. All you have to do is take the beans that have been soaked overnight (as described above) and rinse and drain them 3-4 times a day until they sprout. (Don't worry about the beans drying out. Don't let them sit in water after the first night of soaking.) As soon as they sprout you can eat them raw. While you can eat them any time you please, suggested sprouting times for beans is 3-4 days. If you are sprouting alfalfa and radish seeds, 6-7 days is suggested. After they have reached the desired stage, you can stop them from sprouting further by putting them into the refrigerator, where their storage life is about the same as other fresh vegetables. Sprouting is excellent during the winter when the availability and quality of other fresh vegetables is low and when their prices are relatively high.

The following table gives you some idea of the phenomenal increase in nutritional value you get from sprouting.

Increase in Food Value from Sprouting of Dry Beans

	Vit. B1	Vit. B2	Vit. B3
Mung Bean Sprouts	151%	569%	226%
Pinto Bean Sprouts	54%	369%	483%
Kidney Bean Sprouts	758%	1378%	1401%
Lentil Sprouts*	98%	87%	81%
Pea Sprouts*	-19%	42%	173%
Navy Bean Sprouts	202%	364%	196%

*in order to sprout, you need whole peas and lentils. Split peas and split lentils will not work.

Cooking

Beans as well as whole grains that have been soaked overnight can also be cooked and eaten as is, or served with butter or oil and/or spices. Stored cool after cooking, they can be made into salads, using olive oil and fresh lemon juice and fresh spices such as onion, parsley, dill, etc. Sprouts and cooked beans can also be added to vegetable salads.

Of course, when beans are cooked, they lose nutritional value as can be seen from the following table.

Vitamin Retention in Cooked Beans

Cooking Time	Vit. B1	Vit. B2	Vit. B3	Vit. B5	Vit. B6	Vit. Bc	Vit. B12
15-20 minutes		70%	80%	75%	75%	75%	65%
45-75 minutes		65%	75%	70%	75%	70%	50%
2-2.5 hours		45%	70%*	60%	55%	55%	35%

*imputed

Traditionally, most of the cereal grains we eat (with the exception of rice and millet) are milled into flours, meals, and flakes (e.g. oat meal) before we eat them. I have already stressed the importance of eating whole grain cereals (such as whole wheat, brown rice, etc.). While whole wheat flour is readily available, it is somewhat more difficult to obtain other whole grain flours and meals. For example, it is very difficult to purchase whole grain cornmeal. For those who are interested in making the most of their cereal grains, I recommend them purchasing the Magic Mill [see Appendix]. With this compact food preparation tool, you can make flour from virtually any grain. You can also make breakfast cereals such as cracked wheat and cornmeal. Using my own mill, I can make a number of different cereals for less than a penny per serving.

Cooked cereals are a cinch to make. The following table shows you how to cook a number of different breakfast cereals.

Cereal Grain	Water
1 cup oatmeal	2 cups
1 cup brown rice	2 cups
1 cup millet	2.5 cups
1 cup cracked wheat	2.5 cups
1 cup cracked rye	2.5-3 cups
1 cup cornmeal	3.5-4 cups

Add grain, water, and salt (from zero to one-quarter of a teaspoons per cup of water) to a pot, and bring them to a boil.

For brown rice and millet, stir briefly after they come to a boil and bring to a slow simmer in a covered pot. These grains should not stirred while being simmered. Millet will be done in about 15 minutes and brown rice will be done in about 45 minutes. Rice is more traditionally served at lunch or dinner.

For oatmeal, cracked wheat, and cracked rye, bring to a slow boil and stir continuously until done. They should all be done in about 10-20 minutes after coming to a boil. For cornmeal, stirring should begin as soon as the pot is put on the stove and should continue (for about 20-30 minutes) until it is ready to serve.

These cereals can be served with butter and a natural sweetener such as maple syrup, honey, or sorghum.

Vitamin Retention of Grains in Cooked Cereals and Bakery Products

Food	Vit. B1	Vit. B2	Vit. B3	Vit. B5	Vit. B6	Vit. Bc	Vit. A
Cooked Cereal	80%	80%	90%	85%	90%	70%	90%
Bakery Products	80%	90%	90%	65%	90%	70%	90%

Other Tips

Recipes calling for sugar should be modified to replace each cup of sugar with two-thirds cup of maple syrup, honey, molasses, barley malt, or sorghum to get an equal amount of sweetness.

As your sweet tooth fades, you will find that using one-half cup of sweetener for each cup of sugar will suffice.

Recipes calling for margarine should be modified to replace the each cup of margarine with one cup of butter or seven-eighths of a cup of oil.

Recipes calling for vegetable shortening should be modified to replace each cup of vegetable shortening with one cup of lard, one cup of oil, or one and one-eighth cups of butter.

Your teeth are your most important food processing tool. As elementary as it may sound, it is absolutely necessary for you to thoroughly chew your food and eat slowly to increase the absorption of your food so that you can take advantage of its full nutritional value. If you can't take the time to eat slowly, you're better off skipping the meal until you do make the time.

Chapter 8

Other Needs and Things to Avoid

Inchworm, inchworm,
Measuring the marigold,
You and your arithmetic,
You'll probably go far.
Inchworm, inchworm,
Measuring the marigold,
Seems to me you'd stop and see
How beautiful they are.
Frank Loesser

Quite often, scientists design models to explain their observations and predict what might happen in future experiments. In this chapter, we shall use two of their models referred to as the electromagnetic theory and the atomic theory to allow us to more clearly understand and predict the beneficial or harmful effects of various energies and substances.

Electromagnetic Radiation

Electromagnetic radiation is carried in packets of energy called photons. Electromagnetic radiation ranges from gamma rays, which have very high energy (penetrating) photons and a wavelength of about one-trillionth of an inch, to radio waves, which have very low energy photons and a wavelength of as long as 100 miles or more.

The sun provides almost all of the natural electromagnetic radiation that you receive. The atmosphere which surrounds the earth serves as a shield to protect you from that part of the sun's radiation that would otherwise be harmful. Thus the atmosphere protects you from gamma rays, x-rays, and also filters out a substantial amount of ultraviolet (or UV) radiation. It lets some ultraviolet radiation come through. This ultraviolet radiation has a wavelength of less than 1/60,000th of an inch. With its mildly penetrating properties, it enters your skin and promotes the formation of the hormone, cholecalciferol (erroneously referred to as "vitamin D").

The atmosphere lets in all the radiation with wavelengths between 1/60,000th to 1/10,000th of an inch. Radiation with a wavelength of 1/60,000th of an inch (purple) to 1/30,000th of an inch (red) you can detect with your eye as light. Radiation with a wavelength of 1/30,000th of an inch to 1/10,000th of an inch (infrared), your body can detect as heat. Both nourish your body, one by giving you sight, the other by giving you warmth.

Interestingly, the atmosphere also lets in radiation in the form of radiowaves (with a wavelength of 1/2 inch to 40 inches). While we are currently unaware of the effects of natural radiowaves, it is likely that they not only nourish the body but also are detected by the body internally (which may be good news to astrologers).

Man-made devices expose you to electromagnetic radiation outside the narrow range that you are naturally exposed to. These radiation exposures circumvent your natural defense mechanisms, which would otherwise warn you of overexposure. These exposures certainly do not nourish you and in many cases can harm you. Thus, as examples, you may be exposed to:

Gamma radiation from "nuclear medicine", nuclear power plants, and nuclear explosions, as well as the radioactive chemicals they release into the environment. Gamma radiation can damage the immune system and can cause genetic damage, which may result in birth defects and cancer.

X-rays at the dentist's office, the physician's office, and the hospital for use in diagnosis and "therapy", and x-rays from color television sets and fluorescent lighting. X-rays can also damage the immune system and can cause genetic damage, which may result in birth defects and cancer. In a front page story the December 11, 1985 issue of the **Wall Street Journal** warned, "Each year millions of Americans are getting more radiation — often far more — than they should from medical and dental X-rays." They then go on to quote Dr. John Gofman, former Associate Director of Lawrence Livermore National Laboratory, as pointing out that, "Unnecessarily high diagnostic X-ray doses are signing a cancer death warrant for 750,000 people every 30 years." In his book, **X-rays: Health Effects of Common Exams**, Dr. Gofman lists the chances of your getting cancer from a number of different X-rays routinely given by dentists and physicians.

Ultraviolet radiation from tanning booths and welding torches. (There is also some concern that certain poisons may be destroying chemicals in the atmosphere that help filter out ultraviolet radiation and that this may be resulting in an increased exposure to ultraviolet light.) Since ultraviolet radiation cannot penetrate your body like gamma rays or x-rays, damage to your body from elevated levels of ultraviolet radiation is confined to skin (suppression of the immune system in the skin, skin cancer, and other skin diseases) and eyes.

Microwaves and radar from microwave ovens and close proximity to radar stations and microwave transmission stations. These radiations can cook you on the inside without being detected as heat by the sensory receptors of your skin. Reports of increased incidence of cataracts and other harmful effects have been reported.

Radio waves from television stations, radio stations, and an increasing number of short wave and citizen band communications devices.

Extremely low frequency (ELF) waves generated by diathermy devices, power lines, heating blankets, or any other wiring that runs current close to the body. Naturally occurring electromagnetic activity in the brain has already been observed in this range. Research points to the possibility that the human brain is not only a transmitter, but also a receiver (possibly within the pineal area of the brain) of ELF waves and that these waves may be used for communication within an individual and possibly between individuals. (If you've ever gone to bed with your mate and were aware that he/she, though inactive physically, was still mentally active, you may have already recognized this "extrasensory" perception.) It has been observed that extremely low frequency radio waves affect daily rhythms such as the sleep-wake cycle, as well as behavior and other physiological responses.

In addition to exposing you to types of radiation not found normally, man-made devices expose you to higher doses of electromagnetic radiation within the ranges that you are naturally exposed to. These may also have harmful effects.

Consider, for example, visible light from a camera flashbulb flashed in the face of an infant. While the damage of this short-term high intensity light on the highly sensitive eyes of an infant has not, to my knowledge been investigated, I highly advise that if you feel it necessary to take a picture of an infant, you confine your shot to outdoor shots or indoor shots without the use of a flash.

Radiation is also being used to treat foods.

Gamma radiation and x-rays are used to destroy bacteria and other microorganisms in food that might make food spoil. It is also used to destroy enough of the enzymes in, e.g. a potato, to prevent it from sprouting. In this process, the radiation leaves a witch's brew of fragmented chemicals (such as free radicals and peroxides) which are capable of causing damage far beyond my imagination. In one study, dogs fed irradiated food showed significant decreases in blood proteins. Examination of the food revealed decreases in the contents of essential amino acids and vitamin A, as well as other changes — but no change in taste. As of 1987, foods that are irradiated must be labeled.

Microwaves are used to heat foods. This heating takes place by means of inducing the vibration of water molecules in the food, producing extremely high temperatures at very small points in the food — temperatures far higher than those obtained by thermal cooking of the food. The problem is that this superheating can induce the formation of bizarre chemicals which can cause health problems.

In short, it is wise to take *reasonable* steps to stay away from forms of radiation that you are not exposed to in nature, as well as "irradiated" food products and foods cooked in microwave ovens. In the case of radiation used for medical purposes, you should have serious reservations about using these treatments in all but life-or-limb-threatening circumstances. Those who oppose routine breast x-rays (mammograms) for the detection of breast cancer have pointed to statistics which show that these x-ray exposures cause more cancer than they detect.

Types of Electromagnetic Radiation

Since, according to theory, all electromagnetic radiation travels at the same speed (approximately 186,000 miles per second), the differences in energy of the various forms of electromagnetic radiation is not due to the speed of the radiation. It is due instead to the vibrational energy generated by a photon as it is traveling through space. This vibrational energy varies from about 30 vibrations per second for extremely low frequency (ELF) waves to about 30,000,000,000,000,000,000,000 (or $3x10^{22}$, which means 3 with 22 zeros following it) vibrations per second for gamma rays. In short, it would take the energy of about 1,000,000,000,000,000,000,000 (or $1X10^{21}$) ELF photons to equal the energy of one cosmic photon.

Type of Radiation	Wavelength	Vibrations per second
Gamma rays	1/2,500,000,000,000 to 1/2,500,000,000 inch	$3X10^{19}$-$3X10^{22}$
X-rays	1/2,500,000,000 to 1/2,500,000 inch	$3X10^{16}$-$3X10^{19}$
Ultraviolet rays (UV)	1/2,500,000 to 1/60,000 inch	$75X10^{13}$-$3X10^{16}$
Visible light	1/60,000 to 1/30,000 inch	$43X10^{13}$-$75X10^{13}$
Infrared light (IR)	1/30,000 to 1/10,000 inch	$14 X10^{13}$-$43X10^{13}$

Types of Electromagnetic Radiation
(continued)

Type of Radiation	Wavelength	Vibrations per second
Submillimeter waves	1/10,000 to 1/25 inch	$3 \times 10^{11} - 14 \times 10^{13}$
Microwaves (Radar)		
Extremely High Frequency (EHF)	1/25 to 4/10 inch	$3 \times 10^{10} - 3 \times 10^{11}$
Super High Frequency (SHF)	4/10 to 4 inches	$3 \times 10^{9} - 3 \times 10^{10}$
Radio waves		
Ultra High Frequency (UHF)	4 to 40 inches	$3 \times 10^{8} - 3 \times 10^{9}$
Very High Frequency (VHF)	0.3-3 feet	$3 \times 10^{7} - 3 \times 10^{8}$
High Frequency (HF)	30-30 feet	$3 \times 10^{6} - 3 \times 10^{7}$
Medium Frequency (MF)	300-3000 feet	$3 \times 10^{5} - 3 \times 10^{6}$
Low Frequency (LF)	0.6-6 miles	$3 \times 10^{4} - 3 \times 10^{5}$
Very Low Frequency (VLF)	6-60 miles	$3 \times 10^{3} - 3 \times 10^{4}$
Voice Frequency (VF)	60-600 miles	300-3000
Extremely Low Frequency (ELF)	600-6,000 miles	30-300

Physical Objects

The smallest particles that we are exposed to are protons, electrons, and neutrons. The proton, which has a positive electrical charge, is so small that it would take as many protons to form a grain of sand as it would take grains of sand to form the planet earth. The neutron, which has no electrical charge, is about the same size as the proton. The electron, which carries a negative charge, is probably about 1/10th the size of a proton, and is the smallest particle in the universe that we are aware of. For the purposes of this book, we can consider a neutron as a proton and an electron which have joined together.

The earth's atmosphere is continually bombarded by high speed protons, neutrons, and electrons. We refer to these high speed particles as cosmic rays. Cosmic rays also contain larger high-speed particles composed of protons and neutrons. On the earth's surface, we are shielded from these particles by our atmosphere. However, on the earth's surface nuclear power plants and nuclear weapons produce high speed particles and chemicals (called radioactive chemicals) which break down and release some of these high speed particles.

Atoms

Atoms are the next larger sized particles in your environment. An atom is composed of tightly packed protons and neutrons which form the nucleus, and electrons which orbit the nucleus at speeds so great they effectively form a shell around the nucleus. The diameter of the shell is about 50,000 times the diameter of the nucleus.

The fundamental difference between the 91 different types of atoms which occur naturally is the number of protons each of them contain in the nucleus. This ranges from 1, for hydrogen, to 94, for plutonium. For each proton in the nucleus there is an orbiting electron to maintain electrical neutrality. (Atoms with 43 protons, 61 protons, and 93 protons have not been found as naturally occurring constituents of this planet.) Atoms react with each other to form millions of different molecules. Naturally occurring molecules can contain from 2 to 250,000 atoms or more.

Radioactive Isotopes

Isotopes are atoms which contain the same number of protons but different numbers of neutrons in their nucleus. For example, the predominant form of hydrogen contains one proton and no neutrons in the nucleus, but there are two other isotopes of hydrogen, one whose nucleus contains one proton and one neutron (deuterium) and another whose nucleus contains one proton and two neutrons (tritium).

Tritium is a radioactive isotope of hydrogen produced by nuclear power plants and nuclear weapons. Its nucleus is unstable and one of its neutrons eventually breaks down into a proton as well as an electron which it throws out of the nucleus in the form of a beta ray (high speed electron). Because the atomic nucleus now contains two protons, it is no longer hydrogen, but has transmutated to form a helium ion.

This produces a double jeopardy for your body.

If the beta ray hits important biological chemicals in your body, genetic damage, birth defects, and cancer may result. If you incorporate tritium (as hydrogen) into a biologically important chemical in your body, it will transmutate and damage that chemical, again leading to genetic damage, birth defects, and cancer. Tritium is only one of a number of beta emitters that is a result of man's entry into the nuclear arena. Continual emission of these radioisotopes from "normally" operating nuclear power plants poses a serious threat of increased cancer rates. The build-up of radioactive wastes from nuclear power plants presents an additional problem that has not been re-solved.

Occasionally, cataclysmic disasters occur. For example, in 1986, a malfunction at the Chernobyl nuclear power plant in Russia released radioactive chemicals into the atmosphere. Within two weeks, the portion of these chemicals that had been blown over the United States resulted in beta radiation levels 50 times higher than normal. Radiation levels in Europe were even higher.

Radioactive chemicals also emit protons, neutrons, and alpha particles that can also have harmful effects on your body.

Chemicals

Chemicals consist of atoms or molecules. Naturally derived chemicals do not pose anywhere near the hazards that artificial chemicals do. This is due to the fact over the centuries, humans have developed defense mechanisms against naturally occur-ring chemicals. This is not true of artificial chemicals, most of which were developed within the last 50 years.

In Chapter 2, I advised you to avoid artificial chemicals. In Chapters 5 and 6, I told you how to minimize and avoid poisons in the air you breathe and in the water you drink. I also told you how to identify and avoid overprocessed foods, synthetic foods, and food additives. In this section, I will discuss other classes of chemicals to avoid as well as chemicals which can help protect you against inevitable exposures to harmful environmental factors.

Pesticides

Pesticides are chemicals which are used to kill pests such as insects (insecticides), plants (herbicides), and rats (rodenticides). They have been carefully designed to get around the defense mechanisms of living things and to kill. They are powerful poisons and should absolutely be avoided. I urge farmers and gardeners interested in weaning themselves away from these suicidal chemicals to contact Acres, U.S.A., P.O. Box 9547, Kansas City, Missouri 64133.

Drugs

> "Drugs, being foreign to the body, only by chance evolve therapeutic value and it is more or less inevitable that they harbor some undesirable effects."
> Shigeichi Sunahara
> Tokyo National Hospital

Drugs basically work in two different ways:

(1) You can take drugs as an internal pesticide to get rid of infectious bacteria, viruses, cancer cells, or other parasites before the drug gets rid of you.

(2) You can take drugs to interfere with the normal functions of your body. Taken for short periods of time, these drugs may allow you to get through a crisis with less pain or discomfort. Taken for longer periods of time, these drugs can act to prevent natural events such as pregnancy.

Drugs interfere with the body's natural ability to maintain and defend itself. In the vast majority of cases where drugs are used, the body would have been better off without them. In a small number of cases, they can save lives.

The most helpful thing I can tell you regarding drugs is to stay away from them unless there is good reason to believe that a drug is the only thing which stands between you and eventual death or the loss of some important vital function. If used, the drug chosen should have less serious side-effects than any other drug that could do the job. Even in these cases, the side-effects of some drugs used are so devastating (as in the case of some drugs used for cancer) that the patient may choose death instead.

For those who see themselves as being "on the way out", the use of drugs to treat their symptoms or lessen the pain for their few last years is arguable. But for a person who wants to get their body back in control of itself, drugs are a hindrance. If needed, a drug should be taken for only a short period of time and only in cases where absolutely necessary.

In addition to the above drug problems , we have a semi-legal and illegal drug distribution program going on in the U.S. which is distributing absolutely nonessential narcotic drugs to millions more, bringing a life of misery and crime to the users and those around them. Living in a drug culture, it is difficult for a parent who has become addicted to tranquilizers, pre-scribed for them by their physician, to object when their child starts buying and using drugs that he or she has purchased "on the street".

It is not the purpose of this book to meticulously go through the side-effects of the large number of drugs available. This has already been done in great detail by others. Those interested in this subject should consider reading *Drug Induced Sufferings,* published by Excerpta Medica in 1980, *Cured to Death,* pub-lished by Stein & Day in 1983, and/or D.M. Davies' *Textbook of Adverse Drug Reactions,* published by Oxford University Press in 1985.

The following excerpts from the above publications are included only to give you an idea as to why drugs have not gotten the bad name they deserve.

In *Drug Induced Sufferings,* Dr. Olle Hansson, of the Dept. of Pediatrics of the University of Gothenburg, Sweden stated:

"I am aware of the fact that the problems concerning drugs are very complex. I am aware of the huge economic stakes in the search for new drugs. I am aware of the painstaking control by the medical authorities. But I am also aware of the power of profit and the effectiveness of marketing departments. And I am also aware of the improbability of a drug which is not only effective but also harmless and without unwanted effects.". . .

"The first and most disturbing fact is the existence at the present time of a number of unscrupulous drug companies around the world. This is particularly disturbing as it is quite difficult to find a drug company which does not deserve to be criticized. High esteem by doctors, a famous international reputation, prestige and worldwide marketing are no guarantees for the consumer."

". . . in most countries laws seem to be written for the protection of drug producers, not for the consumers."

". . . in all countries there are unhealthy bonds between doctors and the drug industry. . . . It is not only drinks, dinners, and conferences at home and abroad, and even other things at the drug company's expense, medical journals depend on the income from drug advertisements. The drug industry also exerts influence through direct support to institutions, medical societies and postgraduate education."

In *Cured to Death,* the authors point out:

"Under a veneer of cooperation and goodwill, the drug industry is constantly fighting to extend its spheres of influence. The penetration of the fabric of government, the medical profession, academic and research institutions and the mass media is extensive."

Even defenders of the drug industry admit that adverse drug reactions "yearly afflict millions of people, causing hundreds of thousands of hospitalizations, and deaths numbering tens of thousands".

Protective chemicals

Oxygen is probably the most interesting chemical in the body. In addition to providing the means of burning food to supply the body with the energy it needs, oxygen can be transformed into a free radical called superoxide, which is used by the white blood cells of the immune system to destroy bacteria, viruses, cancer cells, and other foreign substances that have passed into the body. If you are in good health, your body will control the production and location of superoxide. This keeps it under control and prevents it from damaging the body.

Oxygen is also used by the P-450 system of body tissues, especially the liver, to partially oxidize and detoxify pesticides (such as heptachlor), drugs (such as halothane), cancer-causing chemicals (such as PBB's) as well as other harmful substances (such as aflatoxin and caffeine). This system is also responsible for the ability of the body to synthesize hormones (such as cortisone, testosterone, estradiol, and "vitamin" D from cholesterol).

Vitamin A, vitamin C, and vitamin E serve to protect against damage caused by superoxide that might be generated during extremely vigorous exercises (such as marathon runs or long triathlons) or from the generation of superoxide by drugs (such as fluoride) and other harmful chemicals (such as paraquat). They also appear to protect against the formation of free radicals resulting from radiation and radioisotopes. In this context, remember that in Chapter 6, I pointed out that just an average natural food diet would contain about 8 times as much vitamin A and about 20 times as much vitamin C as that recommended by the U.S. National Academy of Sciences. The amounts of vitamin A and vitamin C recommended by the

National Academy of Sciences, while capable of of forestalling obvious deficiency diseases, are not enough to offer protection against the production of free radicals resulting from vigorous exercise, radiation, and harmful chemicals.

While the vitamin E contents of foods has not been determined for many foods, it appears that vitamin E is higher in foods with a higher polyunsaturated fatty acid content. This makes sense because polyunsaturated fatty acids break down easily to form useless and toxic substances and vitamin E prevents this breakdown. The refining of vegetable oils which are high in polyunsaturated fatty acids results in substantial losses of vitamin E, and you'll notice this in your performance. Vitamin E deficiency results in a muscular weakness which can also be brought about by eating refined polyunsaturated fats. This results in membrane damage within (the mitochondria of) the cell and a reduced endurance capacity. This gives you another reason to stick with foods on the recommended list.

In addition to vitamin A, vitamin C, and vitamin E, foods on the recommended list supply you with a number of other substances that are necessary for properly utilizing oxygen. These include iron, zinc, copper selenium, glutathione, carotenoids, coenzyme Q, nucleic acids, hematin, choline, lipoic acid, riboflavin (vitamin B2), niacin (vitamin B3), carnitine, coenzyme A, and a number of other important substances. These substances allow you to physically perform better, strengthen your immune system, and repair the damage done to your body by harmful environmental exposures.

Some foods contain unknown or unidentified substances which are extremely beneficial to your health. Garlic is an excellent example. Among other things, garlic has been found to protect against liver damage, high blood pressure, and atherosclerosis. Garlic also has been shown to have antiviral and antibacterial properties. Examined more closely, it was found that the antibacterial properties of garlic were lost after boiling for twenty minutes. With the knowledge that substances as large as the enzyme, horseradish peroxidase, can pass through the intestinal wall into the bloodstream, it is not unlikely that garlic and other foods on the list actually confer part of their benefits to your body in the form of enzymes, a concept that many close-minded scientists of today will not be able to consider to their dying day. Since many enzymes are destroyed by heat, the possibility that enzymes do play an important role gives you another reason for increasing the amount of raw foods in your diet.

Your body also makes enzymes and proteins to detoxify inorganic poisons that cannot be oxidized. For example, your body can detoxify cyanide using an enzyme called rhodanase. It can also detoxify toxic heavy metals such as lead, mercury and cadmium by making a protein called metallothionein, which binds these toxic metals. The better you take care of your body, the more able your body will be to produce adequate amounts of these substances when you need them.

Problems with Isolated and Refined Chemicals

I already pointed out the harm that can come from the ingestion of polyunsaturated fatty acids without adequate vitamin E. In one study, feeding polyunsaturated fatty acids increased the growth of cancer cells.

Other investigators linked cancer to artificial (trans) unsaturated fatty acids formed during the margarine-manufacturing process.

Consumption of refined sugar as compared to starch has been shown to increase blood cholesterol, triglycerides, insulin, and uric acid.

Similarly, feeding components of proteins, such as monosodium glutamate and Nutrisweet produce problems that never would have resulted if protein from natural sources would have been fed.

In short, fragmenting and refining of food leads to problems that are hard to predict — another reason you should stick with foods on the recommended list.

Heat and Sound

Because atoms and molecules are so much larger and because they move so much slowly than protons, neutrons, and electrons, they are not able to penetrate your body. The faster their random movement, the greater their temperature will be. Your body detects higher velocity impacts on the surface of your skin as heat. In general, your body has adequate defense mechanisms warning you to move away from excessive heat.

If the movement of atoms and molecules is vibratory and synchronous, they will produce sound. The faster they move the higher the pitch will be of the sound they produce, which you can detect due to their vibratory effect on your eardrum. However, the hearing range of an average person is limited to from 20 to 6000 vibrations per second, with a maximum range of from 12 to 12,000 vibrations per second. Since artificial devices have been developed for generating ultrasound (sound above 12,000 vibrations per second) which is above the range detectable by your ear, you can be exposed to the damaging intensity of ultrasound without even being made aware of it. Currently, ultrasound is being used as a tool for medical diagnosis and treatment. While it has not been used enough for me to list the various types of damage that results, you should steer clear of its use for the nonessential treatment of health problems.

Sound waves

Infrasonic	longer than 100 feet	below 12 vibrations per second
Sonic (heard by humans)	1 inch to 100 feet	12-12,000 vibrations per second
Ultrasonic	shorter than 1 inch	over 12,000 vibrations per second

Sleep

In Chapter 4, I pointed out that after balancing all the other factors, sleep should come as a natural result. Experimental results bear this out. According to Dr. Peter Hauri, Director of the Dartmouth-Hitchcock Sleep Disorders Center of the Dartmouth Medical School:

"A steady daily amount of exercise probably deepens sleep . . . athletes and other physically fit people show more delta [deep] sleep than do nonathletes. . . . Mild exercise during the day may also help to start circadian cycling [regular sleeping patterns]."

Dietary deficiencies and dietary imbalances disturb sleep. He points out that ". . . in one study a high-carbohydrate/low-fat diet significantly decreased delta [deep] sleep in humans."

"Many drugs cause insomnia." Among these he lists stimulants, hypnotics, depressants, amphetamines used for weight reduction, monoamine oxidase inhibitors, and contraceptives.

"Caffeine in the evening disturbs sleep even in those who feel it does not."

"The chronic use of tobacco disturbs sleep."

"Poor sleep may be associated . . . with poisoning [by substances] such as mercury, arsenic, and alcohol."

How can you tell if you've had enough sleep? According to Dr. Hauri,

"Ultimately, the yardstick for adequate sleep . . . is . . . a sleep schedule associated with optimal daytime function and minimal daytime sleepiness."

The performance tests described in the following chapter will help you determine the amount of sleep that works best for you.

Vaccines, Antitoxins, and Allergy Shots

> *"Double, double toil and trouble,*
> *Fire burn and cauldron bubble.*
> *Fillet of a fenny snake,*
> *In the cauldron boil and bake.*
> *Eye of newt and toe of frog,*
> *Wool of bat and tongue of dog,*
> *Adder's fork and blindworms sting,*
> *Lizard's leg and howlet's wing,*
> *For a charm of powerful trouble"*
> MacBeth, Act IV, scene 1

These procedures involve the injection of treated or untreated microorganisms, plant products, and animal products into the body. This process circumvents the primary defense mechanisms that would otherwise have prevented them from getting into the blood or that would have destroyed them before they reached the blood.

The purpose for using a vaccine (live, "stunned", or dead viruses and bacteria) is to stimulate the immune system to make antibodies to help fight off infectious agents in case the body is exposed to them naturally.

An antitoxin is an antibody made by an animal in response to an injection of a toxin into its body. The antitoxin is then isolated from the animal and injected into a patient with the hope that the antitoxin will help neutralize a toxin which may be in the blood of the patient. In certain cases, antitoxin injections can save a person's life.

Allergy shots involve taking a small amount of something which a person is allergic to and injecting small amounts of it under the skin. Substances used include extracts of "crude pollen" and "stinging insects".

The question of the effectiveness and safety of vaccines is a real issue. In certain cases where vaccines were given the credit for getting rid of a disease, the disease was already on its way out when the vaccine was introduced. In other cases, such as the swine flu fiasco of the late 1970's, the vaccine is a complete fraud. In this case, 40,000,000 people were vaccinated against an imaginary disease — with a vaccine that wouldn't have worked even if the disease had existed. These vaccinations resulted in an estimated 4,000,000 people who suffered the needless pain and discomfort of a fever, an estimated 10,000 deaths, and additional victims who were crippled by vaccine-induced Guillan-Barre disease.

Here's what the United States Public Health Service, which masterminded the swine flu affair, has to say about other vaccines:

"MEASLES. One out of every four children who receives measles vaccine will have a minor reaction - a slight fever or a mild rash.

"DPT (Diptheria, Pertussis, Tetanus). *Most* children will have a slight fever and be cranky sometime in the day or two after taking the DPT shot. [emphasis added]

"RUBELLA. Rubella vaccine can produce several side-effects. About one out of every seven children will develop a rash or some swelling in the glands within a week or two following the shot. . . . About one out of twenty children and as many as one out of four adults who receive the vaccine will have some pain and stiffness in the joints."

In 1981, the U.S. Public Health Service publication, *Morbidity and Mortality Weekly Reports* admitted that since the rubella vaccine became available in 1969, "The incidence of reported rubella for adolescents and young adults has not decreased appreciably".

Headline articles such as the one that follows should give us further warning. "Federal immunization experts agreed with protesting parents that closer scrutiny is needed of a controversial whooping cough vaccine [used in DPT shots] that has been blamed for injuring and killing a number of children."

Vaccination is a risky business and you should seriously question it before deciding whether or not you or your children should be vaccinated. My choice was against having my children vaccinated. Currently ranging in age from 15 to 23 years of age, they are all alive and well.

Beyond the damage that vaccines can do to you immediately, there are the concerns for the long-term effects that they might have. Vaccinations cause autoimmune responses which can lead to the triggering of the body's immune system to literally eat itself to death. However, in milder reactions, there is the possibility that vaccines could induce life-long allergic reactions.

If a person is vaccinated against a particular virus, their immune system is prepared to identify and destroy the virus before it barely begins to do its job. Staying in the bloodstream becomes an unacceptable hazard for the virus. Thus, instead of multiplying inside the cell, and breaking the cell open to send its many offspring out into the bloodstream to face certain death, a virus is pressured (in an evolutionary sense) into staying inside the cell where a person's immune system can't get to it. In order to multiply without being killed, a virus may be forced to evolve into a virus that attaches to the genetic material of the cell and decontrols cell growth, so that it can reproduce itself every time the cell it is in reproduces. By inducing uncontrolled cell growth, it produces cancer. In short, vaccines would tend to favor the transformation of noncancerous viruses into cancerous viruses.

Vaccinations are routinely given when a baby is about 2 months old. At this age, when the immune system is not even developed, physicians inject 3 different vaccines (DPT) into the baby's body and give it another (polio) orally. By overwhelming an immature immune system at such an early age, it is likely that at least a portion of those vaccinated suffer permanent damage to the immune system. It would be interesting to know what the rate of AIDS for vaccinated people is compared to those who were not vaccinated.

Parents interested in conferring immunity to their children can do it safely by breast-feeding them.

Allergy shots are a dangerous way to try to get temporary relief. According to the Merck Manual, reactions to allergy shots vary "from a mild cough or sneezing to generalized urticaria, severe asthma, and anaphylactic shock. . . . Despite the best precautions, [these] reactions will occur occasionally. The severe, life-threatening ones develop within 20 minutes".

The High Performance Health Program is designed to build up the immune system to allow it to take care of itself without the "aid" of vaccines, antitoxins, or "stinging insect extracts".

Allergies and Intolerances

In addition to being subject to the general adverse effects of poisonous substances in the environment, some people are overly sensitive (or hypersensitive) to specific substances such as certain drugs, cosmetics, foods, plants, animals, and fabrics. These hypersensitivities cause a number of problems such as sneezing, itching, skin rashes, watery eyes, swelling, diarrhea, constipation, nausea, vomiting, stomach pains, weakness, loss of appetite, arthritic pains, tremors, irregular heart beat, photophobia, behavioral disturbances, and hyperventilation. If you find that you occasionally experience one or more of these reactions, going on the High Performance Health program outlined above may get rid of your problem (by taking items like drugs, environmental poisons, and food additives off of your list of exposures). However, there are other exposures that can also produce these effects. These include deodorants, detergents and shampoos, fumigants, paints and varnishes, perfumes, waxes, and cosmetics. Staying away from or limiting exposures to one or more of these substances may relieve your symptoms. Sometimes, it is just one ingredient in a product that causes the problem. By finding a comparable product that does not contain that ingredient, you may avoid the problem. In cases where the product is not essential to your life, you should avoid it completely.

Hypersensitivities to clothing and foods can be largely avoided by sticking with natural fabrics and natural foods.

However, even in staying with natural fabrics, some find they are allergic to wool and that avoidance of wool solves their problem. Cotton appears to be tolerated well by everyone.

Allergies and intolerances to certain foods also present a problem. I have already suggested the removal of milk and dairy products (with the exception of butter) from your diet. In certain instances, milk consumption has been linked to the typical allergic reactions; some have also reported that occasionally, milk consumption may be linked to rheumatoid arthritis, ulcerative colitis, and multiple sclerosis. It has been my experience that dairy products not only cause some allergic reactions, they also make you more sensitive to other exposures (such as cigaret smoke).

Other foods which are often associated with allergic reactions include grains (such as wheat and corn), eggs, finfish, shellfish, and tomatos.

In addition to the normal hazards of drugs, certain drugs (such as monoamine oxidase inhibitors) interfere with the normal breakdown of food components (such as tyramine) and together can have life-threatening effects (acute high blood pressure and death).

If you eat fruit pits or kernels for nutritive value and for the nitrilosides (such as Laetrile, amygdalin, and prunasine) that they contain you should eat them whole, chew them well, and not mix them or let sit with other foods or water overnight. Don't, for example, grind up apricot kernels and let them sit overnight in orange juice. If you do, you will be getting a large dose of cyanide the following morning. This results from the breakdown of nitrilosides overnight. By eating apricot kernels whole, the breakdown of nitrilosides is slow enough to let the body detoxify the cyanide released, allowing you to safely consume the seeds and kernels of the fruits you eat.

Again, listen to your body. If eating beef leads to irregular heartbeats, don't eat it. If you get a runny nose after drinking milk, stop drinking it. If you choose from the tables what looks like the most nutritious food, but eating it depresses the results on your performance tests, try other foods on the list that are also highly nutritious. You don't have to wait until there is a "scientific proof" to back up what your body is telling you. Nutritionally, all you need is the discipline to pull yourself away from eating habits you may have developed and stick with the foods on the recommended list.

Other Exposures to Avoid

Chronic diseases are not so easy to detect. In these diseases there is usually a gradual transition from a normal condition to the appearance of what may eventually be observed as a disease. There is no sharp line distinguishing the onset of a chronic disease. A chronic disease is a disease marked by long duration, by frequent recurrence over a long time, and often by slowly progressing seriousness. This fact in itself often makes it difficult to associate full-blown chronic diseases with their fundamental causes. For this reason I suggest that if you are going to expose yourself to man-made substances, exercise great caution and keep these exposures to a minimum.

Accidents

Many things which are referred to accidents are not. Getting drunk and then getting behind the wheel of a car and injuring or killing yourself or someone else is not an accident. 'Accident prone' people are generally people whose mental attitude is poor and whose level of health is lacking. Either their response time has been slowed because of improper nutrition or drugs (including alcohol); they are not as mentally aware as they should be or their judgement is impaired because of drugs or lack of sleep and other improper health practices; their senses (such as sight, smell, or hearing) are not as sharp because of drugs or improper health practices; or they have suicidal tendencies because of poor diet, inadequate exercise, lack of sleep, or a poor mental attitude.

Accidents are closely related to suicide. In suicide, a person is conscious of the damage they are doing or can do to themselves. In 'accidents', people are less conscious of this. There is more truth than sarcasm to the statement: "Are you trying to commit suicide?" that is asked, for example, of people who are so drunk they can hardly stand and yet still insist that they want to drive home. I am taking the time to bring these facts to your attention so that I can make one simple point: By carefully and conscientiously following the High Performance Health Program, you will substantially reduce your chance of having 'accidents'.

Chapter 9

Performance Testing

The best evaluation of your health is performance testing. It is the only *direct* measurement of your health.

Currently, the field of medicine recognizes absence of disease as a measure of health. However, the health of a sedentary person who has just recovered from a disease is not better than that of an athlete who 'caught' it a week later and is still in the recovery stage. And the health levels of all persons without a diagnosable disease is not the same.

The field of medicine also regards the blood levels of various substances as a measure of health. However, attempts to lower blood sugar levels of some people results in their inability to perform, and, in some cases, causes them to black out. Each person is an individual and their blood chemistries will differ. Even the same person will have different blood chemistries at different times depending upon the activity that person is involved in. While blood analysis may in some cases detect certain diseases, it is certainly not an objective and reliable measure of health.

The field of medicine also regards weight and height measurements as a measure of health. However, an overweight person who gets cancer, who loses weight as a result of having had cancer, and who then gets cured is not in better health as a result of having had cancer. And two people six feet tall and weighing 190 pounds are not of comparable health, if the body fat of one of them is 50% while that of the other is only 15%.

Performance testing is the most reliable way to test your health, and in cases where you have no diagnosable disease, the only way. The best way for you to watch your performance improve is to test it at various intervals. The following battery of tests are designed to allow you to measure your performance.

Time Trials

The most informal means of performance testing is the time trial. You can either ride a bicycle or run a set distance and watch what happens to your time as you repeat the trial. You can see what happens to the time it takes you to run or ride that same distance as you change your diet, begin your exercise program, and start avoiding various poisonous substances in your environment.

Muscle Group Testing

These tests should be performed no sooner than one month after you have begun the High Performance Health Program. They should not be confused with the Basic Exercise Program, which is more extensive than the performance tests.

For the following exercises, use the same weight you used for the Basic Exercise Program and do as many repetitions as you can. After a 45-second recovery, perform the task again. After another 45-second recovery, perform the task once again. Your maximum output for each muscle group is determined from the first set of repetitions. Using the following table, along with the weight you used and the number of times you did the exercise, you should be able to calculate the maximum weight you would be able to handle if you did one lift.

Number of Reps of the Weight You Lifted	For Maximum Weight You Can Lift Multiply Weight You Lifted By
1	1.00
2	1.04
3	1.06
4	1.09
5	1.11
6	1.14
7	1.16
8	1.19
9	1.22
10	1.25
11	1.28
12	1.32
13	1.35
14	1.39
15	1.43
16	1.47
17	1.52
18	1.56
19	1.61
20	1.67
21	1.72
22	1.79
23	1.85
24	1.92
25	2.00

You can determine your first muscular recovery by dividing the number of repetitions of the second set by the number of repetitions of the first set. For example if you did 9 repetitions in the first set, 5 reps in the second set, your muscular recovery would be 5 divided by 9 which equals .56 or 56%. Similarly you can determine your second muscular recovery by dividing the number of repetitions of the third set by the number of repetitions of the first set. As you proceed through the program, you will see the maximum weight you can lift increase and you will also see the your muscular recovery percentage increase.

Leg Curls — [Explained on page 148]

Leg Extensions — Sit down on the end of a leg extension machine with the backs of your knees against the edge of the seat and your feet hooked under the leg extension cushions.

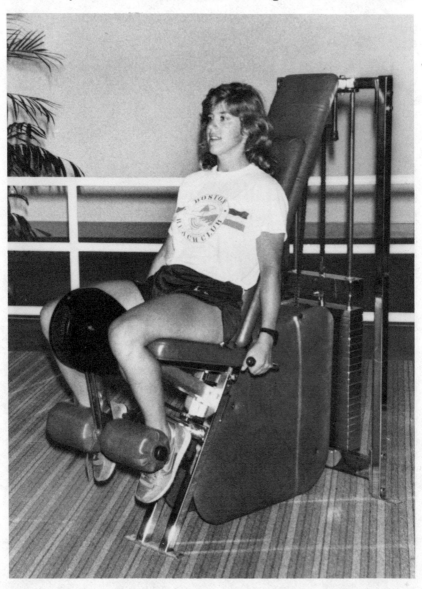

Slowly straighten out your legs, stop, and lower them to the original position.

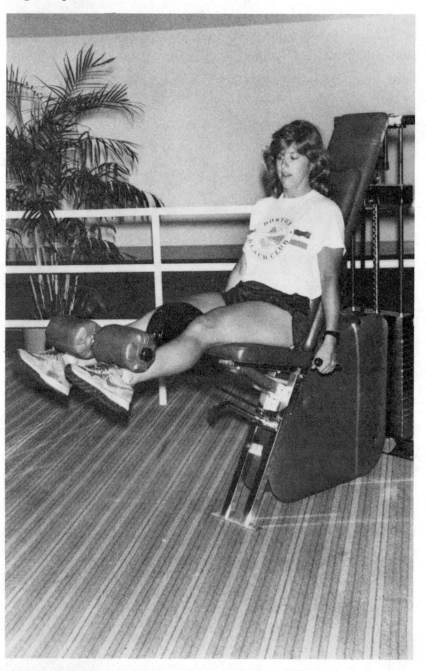

Lat Pulldowns — [Explained on page 151]

Bench Press — [Explained on page 157]

Military Press — [Explained on page 161]

Preacher Curls — Sit down or kneel at a preacher bench and pick up the curling bar with palms facing away from you. Slowly

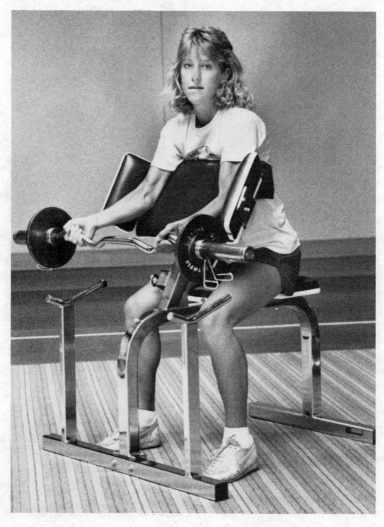

bend your arms until you have raised the bar in a semicircular motion to your chest. At that point, slowly lower the bar back down to its original position.

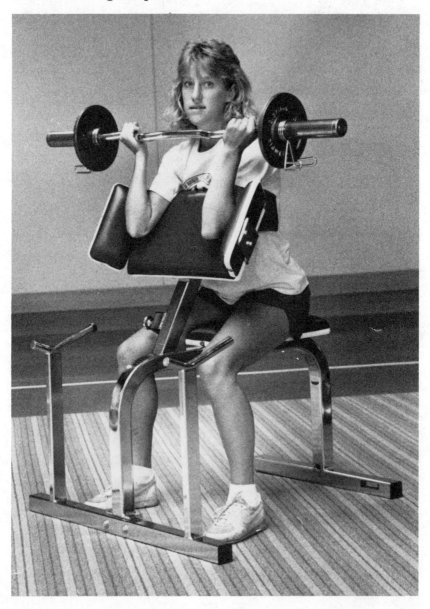

Situps — [Explained on page 176]

Exercise	Maximum Lift	First Recovery	Second Recovery
Leg Curls	_____	_____	_____
Leg Extensions	_____	_____	_____
Lat Pulldowns	_____	_____	_____
Bench Press	_____	_____	_____
Military Press	_____	_____	_____
Preacher Curls	_____	_____	_____
Situps	no weight*	_____	_____

*if necessary the situp bench can be inclined

Recovery of Heart Rate

Before beginning this exercise, take your resting heart rate. Take a jump rope and jump 25, 50, or 100 times. At the end of this time, record your pulse rate at 30-second intervals for 2 minutes. As you continue on the program, you will find that your heart rate after jump roping will return towards resting levels more rapidly.

Time After Exercise	Heartbeats	Heart Rate (Heartbeats X 2)	
0-30 seconds	_____	_____	_____
30-60 seconds	_____	_____	_____
60-90 seconds	_____	_____	_____
90-120 seconds	_____	_____	_____

For monitoring recovery after longer workouts, you can also use this procedure after completing time trials or after doing a workout on an exercise bike.

In addition to tests on muscular performance, tests on the performance of the senses can also be done. For example, you could go into a room with a sign large enough to read easily and continuously dim the light until the sign is no longer visible. After recording the minimum intensity at which the sign was visible, you could then raise the light for ten seconds and dim it down to the minimum intensity at which you were previously able to read the sign. You could then record the time it takes your eyes to recover. Comparing these tests as you go through the program should also show marked after you continue on the program. Unfortunately, while this is an excellent way of measuring performance, the necessary equipment is not available in the average home or health club.

Along with the body measurements outlined in Chapter 3, these performance tests will give you the evidence you need to show you that the program is working.

Chapter 10

The Rewards

In addition to performance testing and taking body measurements – the feeling of vitality, of being alive, and of knowing that your body is on its way to getting into the best shape it has ever been in your life provides a positive way for you to measure the program. In this chapter, I shall present the scientific evidence that shows that the importance of the physical fitness aspects of the program. Remember, the fitness aspects of the program only work when supported by the other parts of the program which include nutrition, environmental health, sleep, and mental attitude. In this chapter, I shall also discuss why this program is the best general program for people who want to lose weight and/or for people who want to avoid diseases, with cancer taken as a specific example.

Importance of the Basic Exercise Program

The Basic Exercise Program was designed to provide a workout combining both aerobic and anaerobic components to increase your endurance, strength, and flexibility in a number of different muscle groups in a minimum amount of time. The exercises used in the Basic Exercise Program have been shown to increase the enzyme levels responsible for aerobic and anaerobic metabolism.

Dr. Jan Svedenhag and coworkers noted that ". . . a tendency to an increase with training was found for PFK [an enzyme important for anaerobic metabolism]."

Drs. Michael N. Goodman & Neal B. Ruderman note that "The following enzyme activities are increased by training: alanine aminotransferase, aspartate aminotransferase, glutamate dehydrogenase [enzymes important for aerobic metabolism] . ."

Drs. Hideki Matoba & Phillip D. Gollnick reported that:

"Physical training induces adaptive changes in skeletal muscle. These changes are localised to the active muscle with their magnitude depending upon the nature, i.e. time and intensity, of the training regimen. The most notable changes are increased concentrations of mitochondria and glycogen . . ."

"Associated with the increases in the concentration of mitochondrial enzymes in muscle in response to endurance training there is also an increased capillary density of skeletal muscle."

It is also well recognized that the exercises used in the Basic Exercise Program increase muscle mass, muscle strength, bone mass, bone strength, tendon strength, ligament strength, and the thickness and resilience of cartilage in joints.

In reviewing a number of studies in his book, ***Applied Exercise Physiology***, Dr. Richard A. Berger notes:

"The increase in strength from weight training is largely attributable to the increase in the cross-sectional area of the muscle. The greater area is the result of more and larger contractile units within the muscle fibers. And, the increase in contractile units is a consequence of protein build-up resulting from increased protein synthesis stimulated by exercise and work-induced responses in hormones and nervous control of muscle."

"As a child grows physically from early age to adulthood, force capacity of the muscles rapidly increases . . . When physical maturation is reached, an increase in muscle force is only provided by overload training."

"Atrophy is prevented by muscle stretch."

"Lifting heavy loads is associated with gains in muscle size. Some of these gains can be attributed to the greater increase in testosterone which is secreted during heavy work."

"Overload training places stress on the skeletal structure just as it does on the muscles. The large pulling and tugging forces on the bones eventually produce structural changes if the intensity of work is high. Although most studies have used rats to show that high-intensity running or overload increases bone girth and density, some observations and studies with humans have shown similar changes . . . Some evidence also shows that bone strength is increased from training and that prior training can accelerate the healing process in broken bone."

"Physical training tends to increase the strength of tendons and ligaments and their attachments to bone so that they can withstand more stress. The exact substances responsible for the increase in tensile strength is not known, but evidence points to collagen."

"In addition to the increase in strength in ligaments and tendons from training there is also a thickening of cartilage between articulating joints."

Aging

Physical changes brought about by the Basic Exercise Program bring about a true reversal of the aging process. In the *CRC Handbook of Physiology in Aging*, Dr. E. J. Masoro points out that

"In a cross-sectional study, it was shown that the fall in muscle mass relative to a total body mass may be wholly responsible for age-related decreases in BMR [basal metabolism]".

Studies show "the occurrence of [an] age-related loss in lean body mass of about 3 kg [7 pounds] per decade of increasing age".

"In most studies [among Americans and Europeans], body fat content expressed as absolute mass has been found to increase-with age until the 6th decade of life".

As a result "Body density falls until the 6th decade of life".

"In American men, skinfold thickness [a measure of body fat] changes little with age over the adult lifespan in the knee and chin, but large increases in subcutaneous fat masses occur in the abdomen and chest during this time while in women there is a marked increase in subcutaneous fat in abdomen, chest, chin, and knee with increasing age, but the triceps skinfold changes little during the adult life-span."

"In the Wajana Indians of Surinam, the skinfold thickness remains constant throughout the adult life-span."

In the same handbook, Drs. N.W. Bolduan and S.P. Horvath point out that

"Active older subjects demonstrate aerobic capacities far in excess of their sedentary counterparts and superior to sedentary young subjects."

"Reaction and movement times for older active subjects are faster than those exhibited by young and old nonactive individuals, and more like those of younger active subjects than either of the nonactive groups."

"Physiological processes known to decline with aging that have been reported to be modifiable by exercise and physical conditioning include cardiac efficiency, arterial distensibility, pulmonary function, and bone calcium."

"The adaptation to physical training which improves performance involved multiple reactions involving skeletal muscle fibers, nervous system, and circulatory system."

"Physical conditioning is associated with the adaptation of

neuroregulatory mechanism to a higher level of functioning."

"Exercise preserves youth."

Is it Weight or Body Fat That You Want to Lose?

The first reaction you might have to losing weight is that it can be done if you can just stop eating. However, by doing this, you deprive your body of the vitamins, minerals, and other factors necessary for your body to perform properly, including its ability to burn up fat. Fortunately, these starvation programs are usually short-lived because your body sends signals loud and clear that its needs are not being met. In cases where starvation diets are adhered to, ill health due to nutritional deficiencies and a loss in lean body mass are the result. Severe cases lead to anorexia nervosa, a level of health so low that body signals can no longer be responded to.

It has already been pointed out that loss of lean body mass, i.e. muscle, is not desirable and that it is not weight you want to lose, but fat. The High Performance Health program is designed to reduce body fat and increase lean body mass. In doing this, your diet is important but exercise is indispensable.

To burn off body fat, your body needs oxygen. By exercising, your body increases oxygen uptake.

To burn off body fat, your body needs iron-containing proteins such as hemoglobin, myoglobin, and cytochromes as well as enzymes. By exercising, your body produces more of these substances.

To burn off body fat, your body needs iron, coenzyme Q, niacin, riboflavin, pantothenic acid, carnitine, lipoic acid, thiamine, and other essential nutrients. By exercising, your body will lead you to the foods that contain them so long as you stick to a natural food diet. Lists of foods high in various nutrients have been printed in this book to help you choose these foods. Performance tests have been described to allow you to fine tune your diet.

To burn off body fat, your body needs your mind. By making the decision to exercise and by exercising, you stimulate your mind to secrete hormones (such as adrenaline, noradrenaline, glucagon, and ACTH) to initiate the breakdown of fats in your body. By actively sensing the rate of your energy output, your mind can regulate the amount of energy your body will burn as fat as well as the amount of energy your body will burn as carbohydrate. On an active exercise program, you will find that your body will burn more fat and less carbohydrate even when you are at rest. This means that you can expect your body to burn about 300 extra calories in fat each day as a result of this change in your metabolism.

To burn off body fat, your body needs exercise. Coupled to proper nutrition and a clean environment, an active exercise program can lead to the loss of as much as one-half pound of fat per day, if necessary.

Cancer

As I pointed out earlier in Chapter 2, your body is composed of a number of cells. In each of these cells there is a nucleus which contains the genetic information which tells the cell who you are, what it is and what it should do. Included within this is the information which tells the cell when it should divide and when it should stop dividing. For example, if you had an operation where a surgeon removed part of your liver, your liver cells would start dividing until they had replaced the part of your liver that was removed. When that job was completed they would stop.

If the genetic control mechanism for turning off cell growth is damaged, the cell will grow uncontrollably until the surrounding tissue prohibits further cell division. Cell growth of this sort is referred to as a tumor.

If, in addition to decontrolling cell growth, the cell is induced to secrete a digestive enzyme into the surrounding medium, the cell will have the ability to digest the surrounding tissues and continue to grow into the space it has carved out for itself. A tumor of this sort is referred to as invasive or malignant. A malignant tumor is what we refer to as cancer.

There are three major ways of destroying or altering the genetic material which controls cell growth and is capable of turning on the synthesis of extracellular enzymes. The first is by means of radiation and radioactive chemicals. In this case what happens is that high energy radiation in the form of alpha rays, beta rays, gamma rays, x-rays, or ultraviolet radiation bombards and damages the genetic material which controls cell growth as well as the genetic material which controls the synthesis of extracellular enzymes. When this is done cancerous growth is initiated.

This damage can also occur if a person ingests, breathes in or is in any other way exposed to radioactive chemicals which get into the body. While in the body, these radioactive chemicals can emit alpha, beta and gamma radiation.

In addition, certain radioactive chemicals such as radioactive hydrogen (also referred to as hydrogen-3 or tritium) and radioactive carbon (referred as carbon-14) can incorporate themselves into the genetic material and upon their breakdown will result in genetic damage resulting in cancer.

The second way is by means of chemicals which interfere with the body's ability to synthesize and repair the genetic material. Falling into this category are drugs, food additives, and other environmental poisons that are dumped into the water we drink and the water we breathe. By interfering with the proper synthesis and repair of genetic material, faulty genetic material is made and again cancer results.

The third way is by means of viruses which get into a cell and attach themselves to the parts of your genetic material. By doing this, they deregulate genetic control of cell growth and the secretion of extracellular enzymes, again leading to cancer.

The High Performance Health Program reduces your cancer risk by eliminating most of the items that produce cancer from your environment. In addition, by means of improving your nutrition and by means of increasing the oxidizing power of your body through nutrition and exercise, the program allows you to more thoroughly detoxify the cancer-causing chemicals that get into your body as well as the cancer-causing substances which are produced in your body.

Your body has a group of enzymes that repair genetic damage and stop most cancers before they start. The High Performance Health Program strengthens this by providing the nutrition which supports genetic repair and by getting you to eliminate environmental poisons (such as pesticides, cadmium, and fluoride) which interfere with genetic repair.

Once cancer growth has begun, your immune system serves as a secondary defense mechanism and tries to destroy the cancer cells. By building up your immune system, and having you avoid environmental poisons which depress the immune system, the program again helps you reduce your cancer risk (as well as other consequences of a deficient immune system such as AIDS, persistent colds, etc.).

Cancer cells thrive on two things: (1) sugar, which it uses as its energy source and (2) the absence of oxygen, so that it can successfully compete against normal cells. By reducing the amount of sugar in your diet and increasing the oxygen capacity of your body, the High Performance Health program gives normal cells the edge over cancer cells.

With the exception of people with rare inherited disorders such as xeroderma pigmentosa and people who already have cancer, I see little reason why anyone who stays on the High Performance Health program should have to worry about cancer.

Chapter 11

Letting The Force Guide You

In this book, I have tried to be quite comprehensive regarding the things you should do to bring your health to a high performance level. Some of you may feel that I was trying to imply that straightening out all the physical things surrounding you would solve all your health problems. This is certainly not the case. I am convinced that there are important parts of our lives that exist in the nonphysical or spiritual world that are essential to improving our health above and beyond the activities and dietary factors that we are exposed to. I am convinced that, in addition to loving ourselves, we have at least three other nonphysical needs: (1) to spiritually and unselfishly devote ourselves to someone else, (2) to spiritually and unselfishly devote ourselves to some ideal, and (3) to spiritually and unselfishly devote ourselves to some god or unifying force in the nonphysical world. I do not believe that entry into the High Performance Health Program for some totally physical narcissistic reasons will bring long-lasting results. Eventually, the person will ask, "For what am I improving my health." If it is to achieve some physical feat or to break some world record, when this task is accomplished or when the person gives up in frustration, what else is left?

However the need to serve yourself, someone else, some ideal, and some unifying entity – and realize the happiness that the

combination of a sound body and a harmonious spirit can bring
– certainly justifies your participation in the High Performance
Health Program. If there is some mysterious junction between
the physical and nonphysical worlds within us, improvements
in our physical well-being is certainly going to influence the
recognition and expression of our spiritual existence.

We each have within us a life force which, during evolution or
some other process, was developed to "watch" over us and lead
us to the things we need until it is drained from us. Ignoring it,
we may leave the "Garden of Eden" it gave us and decide that
the "Tree of Knowledge" offers us better answers. Despite what
this book recommends, if you feel this "force" is advising you to
depart from parts of the program, do it. But don't fabricate some
phoney force as an excuse to alter the program to make things
easier for yourself.

Is the High Performance Health Program risk-free? Certainly
not. If you were to go to your stockbroker and ask for something
that promised an excellent return that had no risk, you know
that in all honesty he/she could not give you anything. The risks
on the High Performance Health Program are not as great as
those in the stockmarket. However, there is a slight chance that
injury could result. You have to weigh that against the opportunity of opening a whole new and enjoyable life for yourself.

Questions And Answers

Question: How old does a person have to be before starting the program?

Dr. Y: With the exception of the Basic Exercise Program, there is no age limit to the participants of the High Performance Health Program. Good food, fitness activities, proper sleeping habits, a clean environment and a positive mental attitude are all important even before a child is conceived. The High Performance Health Program can be maintained throughout pregnancy, with the modification that the weights used in the Basic Exercise Program should be maintained and not increased during the later stages of pregnancy. When a child is born, he/she should be breast fed and started out with a natural food diet free of refined foods such as white sugar and white flour. Growing children appear to have a natural instinct to be active. Nothing should be done to discourage it. Allow and encourage the child to go out and play as much as they wish. School is a real threat to this instinct. It is here where their natural instincts to be active are destroyed and where they learn to tolerate a life of sitting down for long periods of time. When your children go to school, try to get the school to include liberal periods for recess and activities. When your children come home, encourage them to play -- and join in the activities yourself. If a child is into or planning to get into serious athletics, he/she may be able to begin the Basic Exercise Program at an age of 10-12. However, if a child cannot easily handle 25 reps of each of the exercises outlined on page 185

("First Session"), he/she should not begin. Mentally, it is better for a person to start the Basic Exercise Program at the age of 16-20, when they can appreciate the significance of it not being a short-term get-in-shape program, but a life-style that they should continue as long as they want to enjoy a life of good health. If a child as young as 10-12 is allowed to begin the Basic Exercise Program, it should be done as part of a family activity, with Mom and Dad joining in.

Question: Do you really think that a pregnant woman should exercise that vigorously?

Dr. Y: Unfortunately, pregnancy has been looked at as some debilitating disease rather than a normal physiological process. I think I can safely say that the health of mothers and their unborn children have been damaged more from inactivity than from excessive physical activity. It has been only recently, with a greater appreciation for fitness, that sports physiologists have rediscovered that physical activity is not harmful to a pregnant women. In their book, *Exercise in Pregnancy*, Drs. Raul Artal and Robert Wiswell of the University of Southern California state:

". . . current research is corroborating the descriptive and anecdotal studies on high level athletes having no increased incidence of complications in pregnancy and delivery while continuing to train . . . ".

Question: Isn't this program expensive?

Dr. Y: No. As a matter of fact, putting an initial investment into your health will not only pay off in health dividends, it will pay off in reduced medical costs. On the average, getting on the program and staying on it should save you tens of thousands of dollars in medical and hospital costs. Thus, items such as a health club membership and a bicycle are investments well worth the price.

Question: But I already have health insurance. Doesn't this pay for my medical and hospital costs?

Dr. Y: Limited health insurance costs about $100 per month for each adult. This does not even cover the cost of most drugs and office calls to the physician. Even if you are getting coverage at work, it is that much less that you are being paid each month. I have seen some young couples scrimping and saving — buying foods of poor quality — so they can afford medical insurance payments which are either directly or indirectly being extracted from them. Make sure you spend the money to take positive steps to take care of your health before you start putting money out for sickness care.

Question: I am a cancer patient. Will the High Performance Health Program help me?

Dr. Y: The High Performance Health Program was not intended to be used for the treatment of cancer or any other degenerative disease. This is not to say that following some of the advice given in the pages of this book might not help, because it may. The intent of this book is to get to people before they allow their health to fall to a state where it becomes receptive to cancer.

Question: Why do we allow industries to poison the air and water?

Dr. Y: Because these industries provide jobs and because most people seem to be more preoccupied with making money rather than being in good health. Many who have made their "millions" regret that they no longer have the health to take advantage of it. The children of presidents of the dirtiest industries get and die of cancer and their parents suffer the same grief that the rest of us do, despite the fact their very own industrial plant may have been responsible for the child's death. People really don't understand the extremely high toll we pay for environmental poisoning in human health, suffering, and death. If they did, we wouldn't have the environmental problems that we do. Industries can "coexist" with a clean environment. In the short term, we may have to be willing to pay extra for products that are made by cleaner production methods, but in the long run, we will reap the rewards.

Question: Don't we have government agencies that set standards to protect our health?

Dr. Y: We have government agencies which were supposedly set up to protect our health. Having taken some of them to court and won, it appears to me that agency officials are more concerned about protecting their jobs. In two cases, top officials of the Centers for Disease Control (CDC) and the National Cancer Institute (NCI) perjured themselves to cover up the cancer-causing potential of fluoride. The CDC lied to us about swine flu. The Occupational Safety and Health Administration (OSHA) and the International Agency for Research on Cancer (IARC), at the prompting of industry, tried to cover up the cancer-causing potential of formaldehyde. The NCI and IARC joined forces, again at the prompting of industry, to cover up the cancer-causing potential of benzene. The FDA, instead of trying to at least get saccharin regulated as a drug, allows its sale as a food and as a food component telling us that the warning label (on the products it is in) saying that it may cause cancer is adequate protection — as I stand by watching children five and six years old buying saccharinated beverages who can't even read — adequate protection indeed.

Question: What do you suggest for cookware?

Dr. Y: Cast iron or stainless steel pots and pans.

Question: What other food processing equipment would you suggest I consider?

Dr. Y: I definitely suggest that if you don't have one, you should purchase a blender. I also suggest that you consider purchasing the largest mixer made by Kitchen Aid, retail price with vegetable slicer approximately $450 (to find out where to buy them in your area, contact Kitchen Aid, 701 Main Street, St. Joseph, Michigan 49085). Next, I would suggest that you consider purchasing the Magic Mill, retail price approximately $250 (to find out where to buy them contact Magic Mill, 1911 S 3850 West, Salt Lake City, Utah 84604). And finally, I would suggest that you consider purchasing the Champion Juicer, retail price approximately $250 (to find out where to buy them contact Champion Juicer, 6220 East Highway 12, Lodi, California 95240).

Question: Where can I get my water tested and analyzed?

Dr. Y: There are two companies companies that I know of that do fairly complete analyses of water (the cost of a water analysis is $75 to $80): (1) Water Test, P.O. Box 6360, Manchester, New Hampshire 03108 and (2) Water Check, P.O. Box 134, Epping Road, Gates Mills, Ohio 44040. By sending the water analysis along with $15 to Health Action, 6439 Taggart Road, Delaware, Ohio 43015, you can have your water analysis evaluated.

Question: Where can I get good water?

Dr. Y: You can purchase distilled water at a supermarket or have it delivered to your home. Before purchasing it, find out if the bottler is adding chlorine, peroxide, or some other junk to it. If you prefer using commercial spring or well water, get a complete analysis of it from the bottler, including anything the bottler might be adding to it. To have the water analysis evaluated, send it along with $5 to Health Action at the address listed under the previous question.

Question: Dr. Y, when I buy water from the supermarket, I get a plastic taste from the water. How can I get around this problem?

Dr. Y: You can try buying another brand of bottled water and see if you get a taste, you can have bottled water delivered to your home in glass containers, or you can get your own home water purifier.

Question: What kind of water purifier should I get and where can I purchase it?

Dr. Y: I recommend that you purchase a water distiller with a charcoal prefilter. You want to make sure that the distiller is automatic (one that is connected to the plumbing in your home and one that begins distilling water when you need it and turns itself off when the holding tank is full), that the water only touches stainless steel or glass once the water is distilled, and that the boiling chamber is relatively easy to clean. I recommend the following two distillers as being, in my experience, as good as or better than other water purifiers on the market. For table top models, the Durastill model 30J with a CT 4.0 holding tank, price about $600 (for information, contact Durastill, 4200 Northeast Birmingham Road, Kansas City, Missouri 64117); for floor models, the Aqua D Mark II with a 5 or 10 gallon holding tank by Pure Water, Inc., price about $900 (for information, contact Pure Water, Inc., Box 83226, Lincoln, Nebraska 68501). Recently, Pure Water, Inc. has come out with an Aqua D Plus, price about $1000, which reduces or eliminates the need to even clean out the boiling chamber.

Question: How does sugar increase behavioral problems?

Dr. Y: Eating the large amounts of refined sugar normally consumed in the American diet can cause problems in the control of blood sugar. A high sugar meal or snack can produce an over response of insulin which drops the sugar levels to the point that the brain is no longer being properly nourished. As a result, behavioral problems may arise. These problems were recognized as hyperactivity in children by the late Dr. Ben Feingold. In adults, Barbara Reed (Stitt), a former probation officer, found that when inmates were given early probation on the basis that they follow a low sugar diet as outlined by Ms. Reed, repeated offenses dropped off. Both of these investigators gained national prominence for their work.

Question: How does sugar increase heart disease?

Dr. Y: Dr. John Yudkin has conducted research showing that

dietary sugar (which is a raw material used by the body for the production of cholesterol) causes increases in blood cholesterol. Dr. Konrad Bloch, who won a Nobel Prize for his work on cholesterol, showed that dietary cholesterol reduced the amount of cholesterol produced in the body and served as a control mechanism. To understand why sugar is so bad, consider the following. You are a plant manager at an auto assembly plant. One day, someone from a sister plant drops a "whole bunch" of cars (in analogy to cholesterol) in the lot where your finished cars normally go, so you start cutting back on the rate of production of cars. In another scenario, your supervisors pile your materials yard high with raw materials (sugar) for making cars. Your response is to increase production to as high a rate as possible to get rid of the pile and in this process, you end up getting far too many cars stacked in your finished car parking lot.

Question: How does sugar increase tooth decay?

Dr. Y: In two ways. First, its inclusion in the diet deprives a person of the tooth building factors that he/she might have otherwise received had they used their caloric budget more wisely. Secondly, sugar provides a nice food source for bacteria in the mouth which can also lead to an increase in tooth decay.

Question: Do you mean that an organization such as the Food and Drug Administration, which was set up to protect our food and drug supply does not always tell us the truth?

Dr. Y: That's right. For example, consider the following full page ad taken out by the American Sugar Association in the November 12, 1986 edition of the Houston Post concerning a 3-year "study" done by the Food and Drug Administration (FDA).

<u>After an extensive 3-year FDA study</u>

GOVERNMENT GIVES SUGAR

CLEAN BILL OF HEALTH

The article goes on to point out that

"The FDA has confirmed that:
    Sugar is not the cause of obesity.
    Sugar does not cause nutrient deficiencies.
    Sugar does not have an adverse effect on human behavior.
    Sugar does not cause diabetes.
    Sugar does not cause heart disease or cancer."

The falsity of these statements is obvious. As seen in this book, sugar is bound to cause obesity or malnutrition or both. The ability of sugar to bring about other harmful effects such as behavioral problems, heart disease, and cancer have already been discussed in this section.

Question: What can we do to get food companies to make better foods?

Dr. Y: Stop buying their junk food products and start supporting producers of good food.

Question: I have difficulty finding 100% cotton sweat shirts and other clothes. Where can I get them?

Dr. Y: Send a letter to Health Action telling us what types of clothing you are looking for. Health Action Press is currently putting together a catalog of quality healthful products.

Question: Dr. Y, I seem to function better on larger amounts of animal protein than you suggest. What do you advise?

Dr. Y: I advise you to get on the program and take the performance tests to see if you actually do perform better with larger amounts of animal protein. If you do, stay with it.

Question: If you had to list values for the amount of vitamins and minerals a person should take each day, comparable to the way in which RDAs are listed, what would you recommend?

Dr. Y: Anyone, including the National Academy of Sciences,

who lists RDAs is making a serious mistake. First of all, most people can fast for 24 hours without suffering any ill effects. The RDA would imply that these people are suffering from vitamin and mineral deficiencies at the end of the 24 hours, which they are not. Some people will absorb more nutrients from their foods than other people. Depending on the type of food consumed, the absorbability of minerals such as iron and zinc will differ. Some people turn over vitamins and minerals more rapidly. Listing RDAs for the small amount of nutrients that we are aware of gives people the false sense of security that if they can just take these nutrients in pill form, they will be all right. This is not true. However, if the United States National Academy of Sciences wanted to start getting honest with the people in setting up some list of values, their list would look more like the values on the right hand side of the following table.

Nutrient (milligrams)	Old RDA	More Appropriate RDA
Vitamin A*	1	10
Vitamin C	60	1500
Vitamin B1	1.5	5
Vitamin B2	1.7	5
Vitamin B3	19	60
Vitamin B5	4-7	15
Vitamin B6	2.2	7
Calcium	1200	2000
Iron	18	50
Magnesium	400	1200
Phosphorus	1200	2500
Potassium	1875-5625	10000
Sodium	1100-3300	1500
Zinc	15	50
Copper	2-3	6
Manganese	2.5-5	10

*As retinol equivalents

Question: If I stop eating sugar, what's wrong with eating artificial sweeteners?

Virtually every artificial sweetener to hit the market, including saccharin, cyclamate, and Nutrisweet, has been shown to have the potential to cause cancer or the growth of precancerous cells. Just by examining the chemical structures of these substances, a biochemist should be able to predict their cancer-causing potential. However, even if you are not worried about the chance of getting cancer, there are other reasons for you not to eat artificial sweeteners. These chemicals owe their cancer-causing potential to the fact that they cause genetic damage. Thus,exposure to cancer-causing chemicals, in the large number of cases where cancer is not the end result, will induce a permanent alteration of cell function in a number of cells after each exposure. Thus, it may be that after each dose of saccharin or Nutrisweet, you could be losing the functional use of 1000 to 10,000 cells that, in addition, may end up causing health problems by interfering with the proper functioning of other cells.

Question: What's wrong with monosodium glutamate?

Dr. Y: That's a very good question. Years ago, if I had been asked whether or not I felt that monosodium glutamate, which is one of the amino acids comprising proteins, might be harmful, I would have said no. The many hypersensitive reactions that have been shown to occur as a result of the consumption of monosodium glutamate in foods as a flavor enhancer has made me aware that while we biochemists can reliably predict what problems a substance might cause, we cannot predict that a substance is safe.

Question: Why didn't you recommend a specific diet I could follow?

Dr. Y: Every person is different and has different needs. As your activities change, your requirements change. This program gives you guidelines to follow, allowing you to do the right thing while also allowing you to listen to your own body. The flexibility of this program is necessary if you are going to make it your lifestyle.

Question: Should I see a dietitian?

Dr. Y: It all depends who the dietitian is. I am quite sure that it is possible to find a good dietitian. However many of them are not well trained in the area of nutrition or don't practice good nutrition themselves. As an example, I attended the 1987 National Nutrient Data Base Conference. Breakfast was supplied by the conference. Even though this conference was put together by dietitians and others who are supposedly experts in the field of nutrition, the only "foods" that were served for breakfast were sweet rolls, coffee, and a variety of soft drinks including Coca Cola "Classic" and Sprite. And virtually every dietitian in sight was eating this junk. On the basis of this and other similar experiences I have had with dietitians, I would find it hard to give dietitians a general recommendation.

Question: Whatever happened to the basic four food groups?

Dr. Y: There are at least nine: vegetables, fruits, nuts and seeds, grains, meats, organs, eggs, beans, and dairy products.

Question: If I want to get a check-up before I go on the Basic Exercise Program, who should I go to?

Dr. Y: I would suggest that you go to a physician who specializes in sports medicine or a physician who is involved in fitness activities. Make sure the physician is in good health. By recommending a physician of this sort, I stack the deck in my favor that he/she will be less likely to object to your going on the program.

Question: Do I have to be athletically inclined to go on the Basic Exercise Program?

Dr. Y: No, but you certainly will be athletically inclined once you have been on the program for a while.

Question: Why didn't you mention much about canned vegetables?

Dr. Y: In the canning process, 50-80% of vitamins of most vegetables are lost. Vitamin losses in canned tomatoes, which I advised that you might use (in Chapter 5), is only 20-50%.

Question: Are organically grown meats and vegetable products better than those which are not?

Dr. Y: Yes. First of all they should be free of all pesticides, herbicides, and drugs. Secondly, plants grown organically should tend to have a better balanced trace mineral content since the fertilizers used by organic farmers generally contain a better balance of trace minerals. Thirdly, animals on these farms tend to be less confined and as you can see from the nutrient contents of various fowls, activity of the animal appears to be related with better nutritional quality.

Question: What about breakfast?

Dr. Y: Unless you have a low blood sugar problem, I advise that you allow at least an hour, and perhaps two or three hours to pass before you eat in the morning. This period is an excellent time to do a workout.

Question: What workout equipment would you recommend?

Dr. Y: York Barbell. To get information on where to purchase this equipment, write to York Barbell, P.O. Box 1707, York, PA 17405. To get a floor plan for your own private gym, write to Health Action, 6439 Taggart Road, Delaware, OH 43015.

Question: What can you tell me about a calorie-free fat substitute called sucrose polyester?

Dr. Y: First of all, if it ever hits the market, don't eat it. It is a synthetic substance formed by reacting fat with sucrose and is subject to all the problems associated with the other junk fats. It is being developed by Proctor and Gamble, the same company that brought you "Rely" tampons which had been linked to toxic shock syndrome and death, the same company that got the United States Environmental Protection Agency to allow it to use a cancer-causing chemical called nitrilotriacetic acid as a detergent ingredient, and the same company that started the marketing of fluoride toothpastes (a spokesman for Proctor and Gamble has since admitted that a family-size tube contains enough fluoride to kill a small child).

Question: Dr. Y, you presented extremely extensive tables in your book. How can I best make use of them?

Dr. Y: The tables were included for two main reasons. First, to prove that the statements I was making regarding foods and their nutritional value were backed up by sound hard data. Second, they are included as a reference source for you to use when you are selecting foods. While it is important to get as much variety from this list as possible, try to select a good portion of the foods you eat from those listed at or near the top of each table. You will notice that there are a lot of foods on these tables that you have never heard of. These foods are included to allow you (if you wish) to expand the list of foods you eat.

Question: Do I have to follow the entire program to get any benefits?

Dr. Y: No. Everyone will benefit by improving their diet as suggested in the book or by going on the Basic Exercise Program or by staying away from various environmental poisons, etc. However, in order to get the results promised in this book you must follow the entire program. Your question is like asking if it is necessary, when building a square table with a leg at each corner, to use all four legs. Trying to eat your way to good health without doing the other things in the program is like building a table with one strong leg. While it is helpful, it just won't stand up in the long run.

Question: Dr. Y, If my children don't get vaccinated won't they be kept out of school?

Dr. Y: Most states have laws requiring that if you don't want to have your child vaccinated all you have to do is write a note to the school nurse or principal saying that vaccination is against your belief. If they give you any problem, go to your local library and ask the reference librarian to refer you to the appropriate section in the state code and rewrite your note citing the appropriate sections from the state code.

Question: Do I have to stay on the program the rest of my life?

Dr. Y: Yes. Only by making the program your lifestyle can you enjoy its benefits for the rest of your life.

Question: Dr. Y, I run triathlons and marathons and have no problem running long distances but I have a problem running fast. I have been told that this is because I have slow twitch muscles, but that my body is poor in fast twitch muscles and that there is no way to change this. Is this true?

Dr. Y: No. Research by Dr. K. Mabuchi and coworkers from Harvard Medical School and R. Billetler and coworkers from the University of Zurich found that you can increase fast twitch components in your muscles.

Question: Dr Y, it appears that the position of the American Cancer Society is that urban air pollution has nothing to do with lung cancer rates. Is this true?

Dr. Y: I contacted the American Cancer Society and the official I spoke to confirmed that the American Cancer Society's position is that there is no firm evidence to support the claim that urban air pollution increases the risk of lung cancer. As can be seen from Chapter 5 under the section "Where to get good oxygen", there is abundant evidence to show that urban air pollution is responsible for most lung cancer in the United States.

Question: But, isn't it cigaret smoking that causes lung cancer?

Dr. Y: While cigarets are very bad on the cardiovascular system, the evidence which links cigaret smoking with lung cancer is not as iron-clad as it is made out to be. Follow up studies have found that people who smoke cigarets in general have poorer health practices than people who don't smoke. In one study, smokers and nonsmokers were broken down into three groups: (1) those who had high beta carotene diets, (2) those who had medium beta carotene diets, and (3) those who had low beta carotene diets. When matched for the amount of beta carotene (which is a general indicator of vegetable consumption) in their diet, the difference in lung cancer rates among smokers and nonsmokers disappeared for the most part.

Question: I have heard that due to toxic chemicals in the air, water and foods, that it is important to supplement our diet with vitamins and minerals in pill form. What is your opinion?

Dr. Y: The purpose of the High Performance Health Program is to provide the vitamins and minerals you need by the careful selection of foods. If, after consciously choosing foods for high vitamin and mineral levels, you feel you need additional supplements in pill form, try them out. Use the performance tests outlined in Chapter 9 of this book and see if they are improving your performance.

Question: You mention "organic" and "inorganic" chemicals. Can you tell me the difference between the two?

Dr. Y: To understand this, I'll give you a little background in chemistry. About 95% of your body is composed of just three elements: carbon (which has four "hands"), hydrogen (which has one "hand"), and oxygen (which has two "hands"). Plants use carbon dioxide (a carbon using two hands to hold the two hands of one oxygen and its other two hands to hold the two hands of another oxygen) and water (an oxygen with a hydrogen in each of its hands) to form a large number of other substances (proteins, fats, carbohydrates, etc.) which contain these elements. When animals eat plants or other animals, they rearrange the structure of these substances to suit their needs. Because these substances are made by organisms, they are called "organic". An organic substance is one which contains carbon and hydrogen and which most often contains oxygen. Since petroleum products are thought to be derived from living tissues which subsequently decayed, they and the synthetic products derived from them are also referred to as organic. All the substances which are not organic are referred to as inorganic. (In a more pure form, the word organic refers only to those substances derived from living things or from their recently decayed remains. In this sense of the word, the term organic farming gets it meaning as referring to farming where the only substances added to the soil and the elements it contains are organic.)

Question: What is an unsaturated fatty acid?

Dr. Y: In most cases, carbons hold on to each other in one hand to one hand bonds. In some cases, they hold on to each other with two hands. This is called an unsaturated bond, since the carbons could be holding hands with other atoms. In this case, the second hand to hand bond is not as strong and can break more easily, thus making the unsaturated bond less stable. An unsaturated fatty acid is a fatty acid which has one or more unsaturated carbon-carbon bonds. A monounsaturated fatty acid has one such bond and a polyunsaturated fatty acid has two or more. The more of these unsaturated bonds a fat contains, the more unstable it is. That is why, e.g., highly unsaturated oils should not be used for frying.

Question: What is a free radical?

Dr. Y: A free radical is a substance which has a free hand which is not holding anything. It is highly reactive because it tends to grab anything it can get its hands onto. However, free radicals derived, e.g., from foods that have been improperly treated can begin to tear the body apart.

Question: What is superoxide?

Dr. Y: Superoxide is a free radical. It is the first step in the body's transformation of oxygen to water. During this process, oxygen picks up four electrons. As soon as oxygen (O_2) picks up its first electron, it becomes superoxide (O_2^-). In your body superoxide, properly contained, e.g., within white blood cells, is used to destroy foreign substance that get into the body. However, if you are in poor health, superoxide can be formed in excessive amounts and leak out into areas of your body where it can damage you.

Question: You mentioned that consumption of excessive amounts of animal protein was an invitation to obesity. Can consumption of excessive amounts of vegetable proteins stimulate appetite and result in obesity.

Dr. Y: Yes. Consumption of excessive amounts of protein-rich foods, such as beans, can also result in some of the same problems observed with animal proteins.

References

Chapter 2

Webster Third New International Dictionary, G. & C. Merriam Co., Springfield, Massachusetts, 1976.

Thomas Devlin, *Textbook of Biochemistry*, John Wiley & Sons, Inc., 1986, pages 923-927.

CRC Handbook of Chemistry and Physics, Boca Raton, Florida, 1982-1983.

Richard H. Wagner, *Environment and Man*, W. W. Norton and Co., 1969, 528 pages

George L. Waldbott, *Health Effects of Environmental Pollutants*, The C.V. Mosby Company, St. Louis, Missouri, 1976, 316 pages

T. Soda, Editor, *Drug-Induced Sufferings*, Medical, Pharmaceutical and Legal Aspects, Proceedings of the Kyoto International Conference Against Drug-Induced Sufferings, 14-18 April, 1979, Kyoto International Conference Hall, Kyoto, Japan, Excerpta Medica, Amsterdam-Oxford-Princeton, 1980, pages 357-358.

Chapter 3

"Your body is the temple of the holy spirit." *1st Corinthians* Ch. 6, verse 19.

A. C. Nielsen, New York City.

William H. Dietz and Steven L. Gortmaker, "Do We Fatten Our Children at the Television Set", *Pediatrics*, Volume 75, pages 807-811 (1985).

Chapter 4

Richard A. Berger, *Applied Exercise Physiology*, Lea & Febiger, Philadelphia, 1982, 291 pages

Raul Artal (Mittelmark) & Robert A. Wiswell, Editors, *Exercise in Pregnancy*, Williams & Wilkins, Baltimore, 1986, pages 54-55, 152-153, 205-214, 225-228.

Byron A. Schottelius & Dorothy D. Schottelius, *Textbook of Physiology*, 17th Edition, The C.V. Mosby Co., St. Louis, 1973, 590 pages

Peter Hauri & William C. Orr, *The Sleep Disorders*, The Upjohn Co., Kalamazoo, Michigan, 1982, 85 pages

Chapter 5

Thomas J. Mason & Frank W. McKay, *U.S. Cancer Mortality by County: 1950-1969*, DHEW Publication No. (NIH) 74-615, National Cancer Institute, Bethesda, MD, 1974, 729 pages

Webster Third New International Dictionary, G. & C. Merriam Co., Springfield, Massachusetts, 1976.

Arabella Melville and Glin Johnson, *Cured to Death*, Stein & Day, New York, 1983, page 6.

George L. Waldbott, *Health Effects of Environmental Pollutants*, The C.V. Mosby Co., St. Louis, 1973, 316 pages

Jonathan W. White, Jr., "Composition of Honey", in *Honey, A Comprehensive Survey* [Edited by Eva Crane], Heineman, London, pages 157-206.

Kurt A. Oster, "Cholesterol and Coronary Heart Disease", Circulation, Volume 60, page 463 (1979).

D. J. Ross and M. Pteszynski, and Kurt Oster, "The Presence of Ectopic Xanthine Oxidase in Atherosclerotic Placques and Myocardial Tissues, *Proceedings of the Society of Experimental Biology and Medicine*, Volume 144, p. 523.

D. J. Ross, et al., "Atherogenesis Caused by Bovine Xanthine Oxidase-Containing Liposomes", New York Academy of Sciences Conference on Liposomes and their Use in Biology and Medicine, September 1977.

Toxicants Occurring Naturally in Foods, 2nd Edition, National Academy of Sciences, Washington, D.C. 1973, 624 pages

Thomas M. Devlin, *Textbook of Biochemistry*, 2nd Edition, John Wiley & Sons, New York, 1986, 1016 pages

Chapter 6

John Yiamouyiannis, *Fluoride the Aging Factor*, 2nd Edition, Health Action Press, Delaware, Ohio, 1986, 204 pages

Peter Hauri & William C. Orr, *The Sleep Disorders*, The Upjohn Co., Kalamazoo, Michigan, 1982, 85 pages

Raul Artal & Robert A. Wiswell, Editors, *Exercise in Pregnancy*, Williams & Wilkins, Baltimore, 1986, pages 54-55, 152-153, 205-214, 225-228.

Richard A. Berger, *Applied Exercise Physiology*, Lea & Febiger, Philadelphia, 1982, 291 pages

Byron A. Schottelius & Dorothy D. Schottelius, *Textbook of Physiology*, 17th Edition, The C.V. Mosby Co., St. Louis, 1973, 590 pages

Banesh Hoffman, *Albert Einstein, Creator & Rebel*, 1972.

(reduced estrogen) in *Exercise in Pregnancy*, edited by Raul Artel and Robert A. Wiswell, Williams and Wilkins, Baltimore, 1986, page 54.

Recommended Dietary Allowances, 9th Revised Edition, Committee on Dietary Allowances, Food and Nutrition Board, Divison of Biological Sciences, Assembly of Life Sciences, National Research Council, National Academy of Sciences, Washington, D.C., 1980, 185 pages

Thomas M. Devlin, *Textbook of Biochemistry*, 2nd Edition, John Wiley & Sons, New York, 1986, pages 923-927.

Nutrient Data Base for Standard Reference, Full Version for Microcomputers (Macintosh version), U. S. Department of Agriculture, 1984 (March 13, 1987).

Annabel L. Merrill & Bernice K. Watt, *Energy Value of Foods Basis and Derivation*, U.S. Department of Agriculture, Agriculture Handbook No. 74, Slightly revised February 1973, 105 pages

Richard G. Allison and Frederick R. Senti, *A Perspective on the Application of the Atwater System of Food Energy Assessment*, Life Sciences Research Office, FASEB, Bethesda, MD, 1983, 59 pages

Composition of Foods: Beef Products, U.S. Department of Agriculture, Agriculture Handbook Number 8-13.

Composition of Foods: Legumes and Legume Products, U.S. Department of Agriculture, Agriculture Handbook Number 8-16.

Bowes and Church's Food Values of Portions Commonly Used, J. B. Lippincott Co., Philadelphia, 1985, 242 pages

A. Strocchi and R. T. Holman, "Analysis of Fatty Acids in Butterfat", Riv. Ital. Sostanze, Volume 48, pages 617-628

(1971).

C. Hitchcock and B. W. Nichols, *Plant Lipid Biochemistry*, Academic Press, New York, 1971, pages 74-79.

Pamela A. Anderson and Howard W. Sprecher, "Omega-3 Fatty Acids in Nutrition and Health", *Dietetic Currents (Ross)*, Volume 14, No. 2, pages 7-12 (1987).

Norman Salem, Hee-Yong Kim, and James A. Yergey, "Docosahexaenoic Acid: Membrane Function and Metabolism", *Health Effects of Polyunsaturated Fatty Acids in Seafoods*, Academic Press, New York, 1986, pages 263-317.

Artemis P. Simopoulos and Norman Salem, "Purslane: A terrestrial Source of Omega-3 Fatty Acids", *New England Journal of Medicine*, Volume 315, page 833 (1986).

Richard A. Berger, *Applied Exercise Physiology*, Lea & Febiger, Philadelphia, 1982, 291 pages

Raul Artal & Robert A. Wiswell, Editors, *Exercise in Pregnancy*, Williams & Wilkins, Baltimore, 1986, pages 54-55, 152-153, 205-214, 225-228.

Oded Bar-Or, *Pediatric Sports Medicine for the Practioner*, Springer-Verlag, New York.

Chapter 7

Robert S. Harris and Endel Karmas, in *Nutritional Evaluation of Food Processing*, AVI, Westport, CT, 1975, page vii.

Sharon Garland, "Provisional Table on Percent Retention of Nutrients in Food Preparation", U.S. Department of Agriculture, Agriculture Handbook, Slightly revised April 1984.

Chapter 8

Van Nostrand's Scientific Encyclopedia, Sixth Edition, Van

Nostrand Rheinhold, New York City, 1983, page 1061

John Kraus, *Our Cosmic Universe*, Cygnus-Quasar Books, 1980, 283 pages

"Faulty X-ray Devices, Untrained Operators Overdose U.S. Patients," *Wall Street Journal*, Dec. 11, 1985, pages 1, 26.

John W. Gofman and Egan O'Connor, *X-Rays: Health Effects of Common Exams, 1986.*

"Research Shows Sunburns May Alter Immune System Responses", *Delaware Gazette*, July 16,1985, page 14.

H. Mikolajczyk, "Radio Frequency Radiation", in *Encyclopedia of Occupational and Health Safety* [Luigi Parmegianni, Editor], International Labor Organization, 1983, Volume 2, pages 1873-1879

George M. Wilkenning, "Nonionizing Radiation" in *Patty's Industrial Hygiene and Toxicology*, Volume I, pages 359-440 (1978).

Sol M. Michaelson, "Nonionizing Electromagnetic Radiation" in *Patty's Industrial Hygiene and Toxicology*, Volume IIIB, pages 579-651 (1978).

R. Wever, "ELF-effects on Human Circadian Rhythms," *ELF and VLF Electromagnetic Field Effects* [M.A. Persinger, Editor], Plenum Pub., New York, pages 101-144 (1974).

Robert I. Kavet and Robert S. Banks, "Emerging Issues in Extremely Low Frequency and Magnetic Field Health Research", *Environmental Research*, Volume 39, 386-404 (1986).

R. A. Jaffee, R.D. Phillips, and W. T. Kane, "Effects of Chronic Exposure to a 60-Hz Electric Field on Synaptic Transmission and Peripheral Nerve Function in the Rat", in *Biological Effects of ELF Electromagnetic Fields* [R. D. Phillips, et al. Editors], Technical Information Center, 1976, pages 277-296.

R. J. Spiegel, J. S. Ali, J. F. Peoples, and W. T. Joines, "Measurement of Small Mechanical Vibrations of Brain Tissue Exposed to Extremely Low Frequency Electric Fields", *Bioelectromagnetics*, Volume 7, pages 295-306 (1986).

J. W. Lookard Jr., E. L. Carstensen, and T. Morris, Inhibition of Respiration in Cats by ELF Electric Fields", *IEEE Trans. Biomed. Eng.*, Volume 33, pages 473-476 (1986).

John W. Gofman, *Radiation and Human Health*, Sierra Club Books, San Francisco, 1981, page 235.

Robert S. Harris and Endel Karmas, in *Nutritional Evaluation of Food Processing*, AVI, Westport, CT, 1975, pages 393-411.

K. Smid, J. Dvorak, and J. Hrusovsky, "The Effect of Feeds with Ionizing Irradiation on Biochemical Indicators of the Nutritional Value of Energy Nutrients," *Vet. Med.*, Volume 30, pages 531-541 (1985).

Chernobyl Federal Response Cum. ERAMS Air Report (last revised on May 21, 1986 at 9:30 A.M.) 108 pages

Marvin H. Dickerson and Thomas J. Sullivan, *ARAC Response to the Chernobyl Reactor Accident*, Lawrence Livermore National Laboratory, UCID-20834, July 1986, 33 pages

Shigeichi Sunahara in Takemune Soda, Editor, Drug *Induced Sufferings*, , Excerpta Medica, Oxford, 1980, page 5.

H. Jick, "Drugs — Remarkably Nontoxic", *New England Journal of Medicine*, Volume 291, page 84 (1974)

Olle Hansson in *Drug Induced Sufferings* (Takemune Soda, Editor), Excerpta Medica, Oxford, 1980, pages 21, 22, 25,

Arabella Melville and Glin Johnson, *Cured to Death*, Stein

& Day, New York, 1983, pages 5-6.

Shaun D. Black and Minor J. Coon, "P-450 Cytochromes: Structure and Function", unpublished, 1986, 59 pages

Youssef Hatefi, "The Mitochondrial Electron Transport and Oxidative Phosphorylation System", *Annual Review of Biochemistry*, Volume 54, pages 1015-1069 (1985).

Pathology of Oxygen (Anna P. Auter, Editor), Academic Press, New York, 1982, 368 pages

Biology of Vitamin E (Ciba Foundation Symp. 101), Pittman (London), 1983, 260 pages

P.S. Nikov and M.S. Parzian, "Various Aspects of the Effect of Nutritional Factors on the Metabolism and Biological Action of Aflatoxin B1 in the Rat Liver," *Vopr. Med. Khim.*, Volume 4, pages 94-99 (1985).

V. Yu. Akhundov, A.A. Aliev, A.E. Kulgavin and T.N. Sarina, "Effect of Combined and Separate Exogenous Vitamin Administration on the Level of Chromosomal Aberrations Induced by Sodium Fluoride in Rats in Subacute Experiments," *Izv. Akad. Nauk Az. SSR, Ser. Biol. Nauk.*, Volume 31, pages 3-5 (1981).

Sh. S. Tazhibaev, A.A. Mamyrbaev and F.Kh. Takhtaev, "Effect of the Combined Action of Hydrogen Fluoride and Phosphine on the Structural and Functional Properties of the Sarcoplasmic Reticulum Membranes of the Myocardium with Nutrition of Varying Character," *Vopr. Pitan.*, No. 5, pages 40-43 (1985).

T. Javor, F. Tarnok, T. Past and S. Nagy, "Cytoprotective Effect of Free Radical Scavengers Against Mucosal Damage Produced by Different Antirheumatic Drugs," *Int. J. Tissue React.*, Volume 8, pages 35-40 (1986).

M.Y. Morgan, "Hepatoprotective Agents in Alcoholic Liver Disease," *Acta Med. Scand.*, Volume 703, pages 225-233

(1985).

Z.W. Zhou, Z.G. Liu, C.S. Dai and L.R. Ma, "Studies on Antiradiation Drugs: Synthesis of Amino-lipoates and Related Compounds," *Yao Hsueh Hsueh Pao.*, Volume 19, pages 742-747 (1984).

K. Bodo and G. Benko, "The Effect of Radioprotective Compounds on Brain Serotonin Metabolism of Irradiated Experimental Animals," *Radiobiol. Radiother. (Berl)*, Volume 26, pages 589-597 (1985).

N.F. Sheard, J.A. Tayek, B.R. Bistrian, G.L. Blackburn and S.H. Zeisel, "Plasma Choline Concentration in Humans Fed Parenterally," *Am. J. Clin. Nutr.*, Volume 43, pages 219-224 (1986).

J. Wilson and K. Lorenz, "Biotin and Choline in Foods— Nutritional Importance and Methods of Analysis: A Review," *Food Chem.*, Volume 4, pages 115-129 (1971).

J. Stanisz, B.M. Wice and D.E. Kennell, "Serum Factors that Stimulate Fatty Acid Oxidation: Physiological Specificity," *J. Cell Physiol.*, Volume 126, pages 141-146 (1986).

S. Nakagawa, S. Yoshida, Y. Hirao, S. Kasuga and T. Fuwa, "Cytoprotective Activity of Components of Garlic, Ginseng and Ciuwjia on Hepatocyte Injury Induced by Carbon Tetrachloride in Vitro," *Hiroshima J. Med. Sci.*, Volume 34, pages 303-309 (1985).

A. Rashid and H.H. Khan, "The Mechanism of Hypotensive Effect of Garlic Extract," *JPMA*, Volume 35, pages 357-362 (1985).

J.K. Mand, P.P. Gupta, G.L. Soni and R. Singh, "Effect of Garlic on Experimental Atherosclerosis in Rabbits," *Indian Heart J.*, Volume 37, pages 183-188 (1985).

Y. Tsai, L.L. Cole, L.E. Davis, S.J. Lockwood, V. Simmons and G.C. Wild, "Antiviral Properties of Garlic: In Vitro

Effects on Influenza B, Herpes Simplex and Coxsackie Viruses," *Planta Med.*, No. 5, pages 460-461 (1985).

H.C. Chen, M.D. Chang and T.J. Chang, "Antibacterial Properties of Some Spice Plants Before and After Heat Treatment," *Chung Hua Min Kuo Wei Sheng Wu Chi Mien I Hsueh Tsa Chih*, Volume 18, pages 190-195 (1985).

B.D. Roebuck, D.S. Longnecker, K.J. Baumgartner and C.D. Thron, "Carcinogen-Induced Lesions in the Rat Pancreas: Effects of Varying Levels of Essential Fatty Acid," *Cancer Res.*, Volume 45, pages 5252-5256 (1985).

Dean H. Hamer, "Metallothionein," *Ann. Rev. Biochem.*, Volume 55, pages 913-951 (1986).

Mary G. Enig, Robert J. Munn, and Mark Keeney, "Dietary Fat and Cancer Trends—A Critque," *Federation Proceedings*, Volume 37, pages 2215-2220 (1978).

Beatrice Trum Hunter, *The Great Nutrition Robbery*, Charles Scribner's Sons, New York, 1978, pages 67-70, 209-212.

S. Reiser, "Effect of Dietary Sugars on Metabolic Risk Factors Associated with Heart Disease," *Nutr. Health*, Volume 3, pages 203-216 (1985).

L.S. Hentges, D.C. Beitz, N.L. Jacobson and A.D. McGilliard, "Cholesterol Transport and Uptake in Miniature Swine Fed Vegetable and Animal Fats and Proteins. 2. LDL Uptake and Cholesterol Distribution in Tissues," *Lipids*, Volume 20, pages 757-764 (1985).

McGraw Hill Encyclopedia of Science and Technology, Volume 12, pages 656-666 (1982).

Peter Hauri, *The Sleep Disorders*, Upjohn, 1982, 85 pages

Ivan Illich, *Medical Nemesis*, Pantheon Books, New York, 1976, page 16.

DHEW Publication No, (OS) 77-50058 (10/77).

Morbidity and Mortality Weekly Report, February 6, 1981

Delaware Gazette, May 13, 1986

Merck Manual, 13th Edition, Merck Sharp & Dohme Research Laboratories, 1977, pages 228-229.

Ranjit Kumar Chandra, *Food Intolerance*, Elsevier, New York, 1984, 260 pages

R. St. C. Bareston and M. H. Lessof in *Clinical Reactions to Food* [M. H. Lessof, editor], John Wiley and Sons, Chichester, 1983, pages 20-22.

Dean Burk, Personal Communication, June 13, 1987.

Chapter 10

Jan Svedenhag, Jan Henrikson & Anders Juhlin-Dannfelt, "B-Adrenergic Blockade and Training in Human Subjects: Effects on Muscle Metabolic Capacity," *American Journal of Physiology*, Volume 247 (Endocrinol. Metab. 10): E305-311 (1984).

Michael N. Goodman & Neal B. Ruderman, "Influence of Muscle Use on Amino Acid Metabolism," Exercise and Sport Sciences Reviews (R. L. Terjung, Ed.), Vol. 10, p. 13 (1982).

Hideki Matoba & Philip D. Gollnick, "Response of Skeletal Muscle to Training," *Sports Medicine* Volume 1, pages 240-251 (1984).

Richard A. Berger, *Applied Exercise Physiology*, Lea & Febiger, Philadelphia, 1982, 291 pages 17, 22, 24, 25.

T. Reilly, *Sports Fitness and Sports Injuries*, Faber & Faber (London) 1981..

CRC Handbook of Physiology in Aging [Edward J. Masoro, Editor], CRC Press Inc., Boca Raton, Florida, 1981.

Index

About the Author

Dr. Yiamouyiannis received his B.S. in biochemistry from the University of Chicago and his Ph.D. from the University of Rhode Island. Since then he has served as a post-doctoral fellow at the Western Reserve University School of Medicine, a biochemical editor for the American Chemical Society, science director of the National Health Federation, president of the Safe Water Foundation, and director of Health Action. He has spent over 20 years working on the High Performance Health Program, using his children and himself as the guinea pigs. The results have been amazing. Each one of his six children are high performance athletes. Medical costs for his family have been less than $5 per person per year. And he has developed a program where adults can develop a higher level of performance than they have ever experienced in their life. In his book, Dr. Yiamouyiannis shares this program with you and helps you find the way to High Performance Health.

Professional models were purposely not used in this book. Instead, the author used family members to help the reader evaluate the condition of those who are on the program. On the following pages are a picture of the remainder of the family and a picture of Carmen Yiamouyiannis crossing the finish line in first place for women 21 years of age or under in the 1984 Ironman Triathlon international competition in Hawaii. More important than her place, look at the expression on her face and the absence of stress that so often is seen on other competitors in this grueling race.

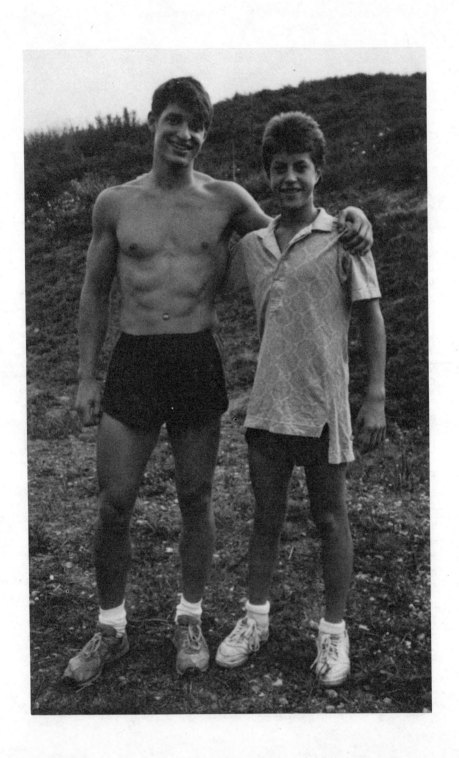

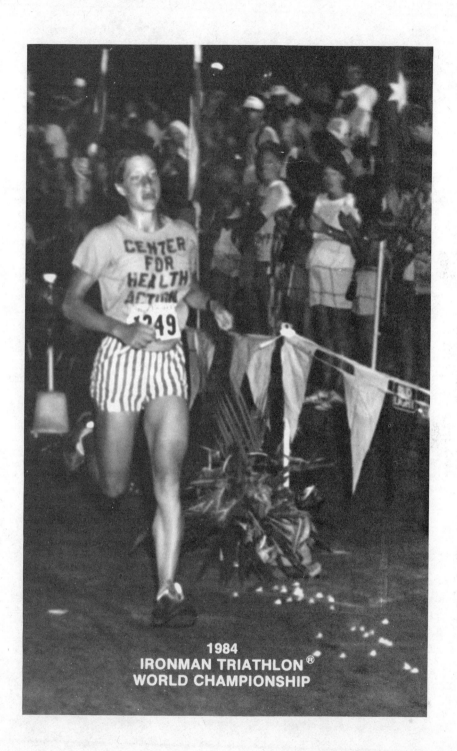

1984
IRONMAN TRIATHLON®
WORLD CHAMPIONSHIP